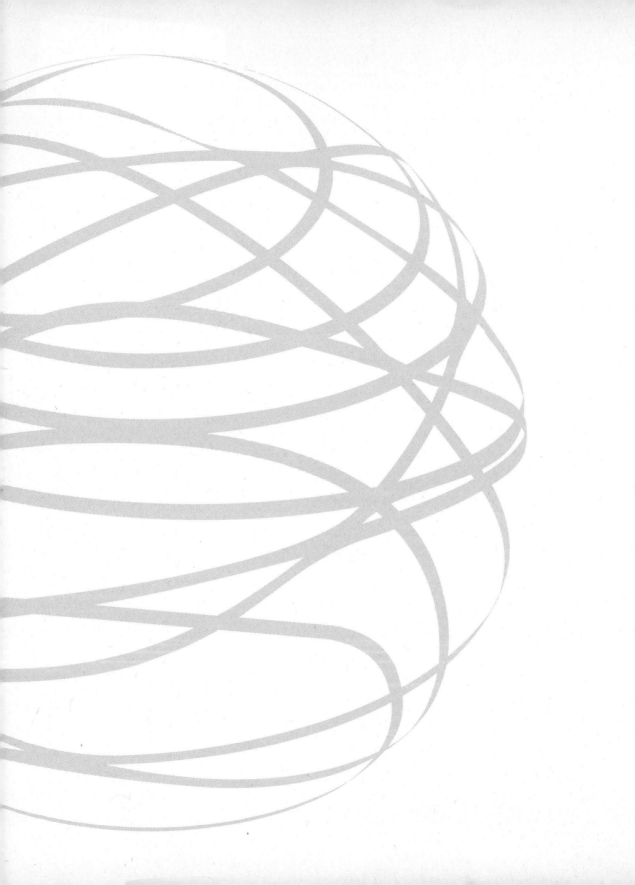

ENERGY WORK

FOR THE EVERYDAY TO ELITE

ATHLETE

About the Author

Cyndi Dale (Minneapolis, MN) is an internationally renowned author, speaker, healer, and business consultant. She is president of Life Systems Services, through which she has conducted over 70,000 client sessions and presented training classes throughout Europe, Asia, and the Americas. Cyndi is the author of numerous books, including *Llewellyn's Complete Book of Chakras*, *Advanced Chakra Healing*, *The Spiritual Power of Empathy*, and *Awaken Clairvoyant Energy*.

ENERGY WORK

FOR THE EVERYDAY TO ELITE
ATHLETE

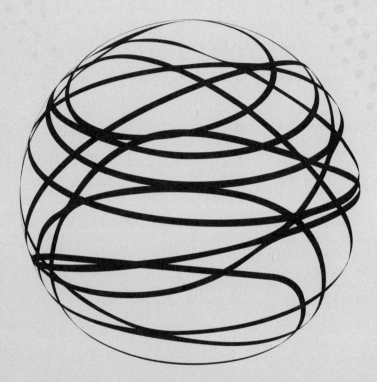

HOW TO ACHIEVE OPTIMAL SPORTS PERFORMANCE
CYNDI DALE

Llewellyn Publications
WOODBURY, MINNESOTA

FIRST EDITION
First Printing, 2023

Book design by Rebecca Zins
Cover design by Kevin R. Brown
Figurative illustrations on pages 32, 55, 58, 124, 196, and in the color insert are by Mary Ann Zapalac and on pages 62, 84, 90, 122, and 126 by the Llewellyn Art Department

Llewellyn is a registered trademark of Llewellyn Worldwide Ltd.

Library of Congress Cataloging-In-Publication Data
Names: Dale, Cyndi, author.
Title: Energy work for the everyday to elite athlete : how to achieve
  optimal sports performance / Cyndi Dale.
Description: First edition. | Woodbury, Minnesota : Llewellyn Publications,
  [2023] | Includes bibliographical references and index. | Summary: "This
  comprehensive guide teaches athletes of any level how to apply subtle
  energy concepts and practices to benefit sports performance and includes
  58 exercises and a special chapter for coaches"—Provided by publisher.
Identifiers: LCCN 2022054375 (print) | LCCN 2022054376 (ebook) | ISBN
  9780738770666 (paperback)
Subjects: LCSH: Physical education and training. | Athletes—Training of. |
  Sports—Physiological aspects. | Energy metabolism.
Classification: LCC GV711.5 .D35 2023 (print) | LCC GV711.5 (ebook) | DDC
  796.071—dc23/eng/20221219
LC record available at https://lccn.loc.gov/2022054375
LC ebook record available at https://lccn.loc.gov/2022054376

Llewellyn Publications
A Division of Llewellyn Worldwide Ltd.
2143 Wooddale Drive
Woodbury MN 55125-2989

www.llewellyn.com
Printed in the United States of America

You can lose when you outscore somebody in a game, and you can win when you are outscored. Make your effort to do the very best you can.

—John Wooden, a successful basketball coach with a 27-year legacy at UCLA, in *Life Wisdom*

CONTENTS

List of Exercises & Tips ... xi

Foreword by Ryan Morris ... xv

Foreword by Dr. Nitin Bhatnagar ... xvii

Introduction ... 1

Part 1: Get Ready and Set!

1 How Energetics Boosts Sports of All Sorts, 9

2 Energy as the Problem and the Antidote, 29

3 Subtle Structures for Changing Energy, 51

4 Get-Set Techniques: Your Basic Energy Tool Kit, 67

Part 2: Energy Work for the Athlete

5 The P's Leading to Performance, 101

6 The Keys to Mechanics, 111

7 Athletic Preparation, 145

8 Injury Prevention and Care—and Speedy Recovery, 169

9 Game Day, 189

10 Dealing with Ups and Downs, 203

11 Special Chapter for Coaches, 229

Conclusion ... 253

Recommended Resources ... 255

Bibliography ... 265

Index ... 273

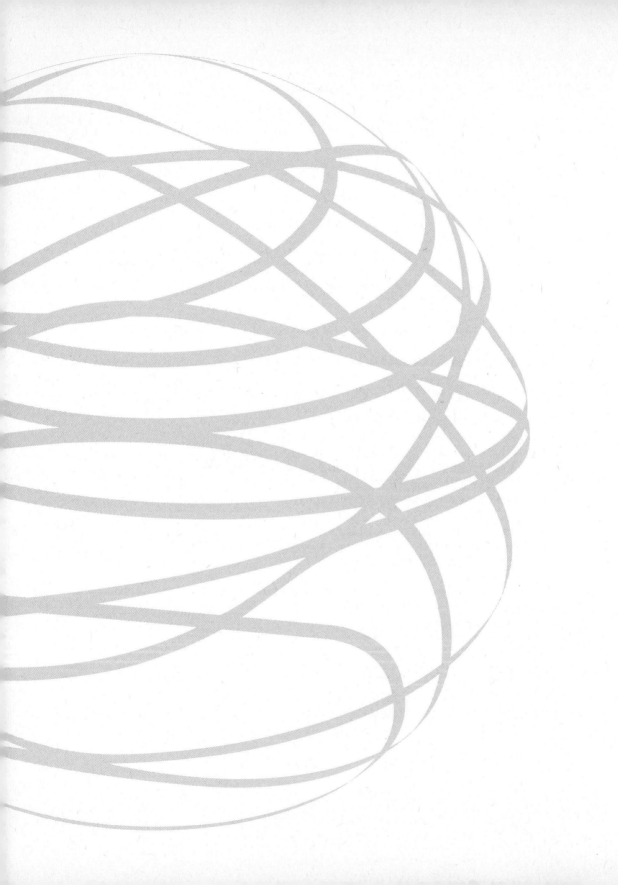

EXERCISES & TIPS

1   The Four-Six Breath   26

2   Finding a Block   30

3   Are You Dealing with Trauma?   35

4   Sensing a Traumatic Block   48

5   A Two-Day Focus   65

6   Sports Spirit   70

7   The Streams   74

8   Gaining Spiritual Guidance   78

9   Chain-Lock   78

10   Visualization   79

11   Applied Kinesiology with a Partner   81

12   Applied Kinesiology on Your Own   82

13   Applied Kinesiology to Use the Body's Flow   82

14   Go Gamma Gameline   86

15   Energy Analysis and Healing   86

16   Emotional Freedom Technique (EFT)   91

17   Hands-On Healing   94

18   Quick Absentee Healing   94

19   Programming Your Water   97

20   Grounding for Pulling In and Pushing Off   132

21   Establish a Vivaxis Grounding Branch   133

22   Adding New Frequencies   134

23   Stabilizing Your Center of Gravity   135

24   Through the Ming Men Doorway   137

25   Clearing and Strengthening the Three Cardinal Planes
of the Subtle Body   138

26   Gamma Gameline for Mechanics   141

27   Quick Shot of Velocity   142

28   Subtly Sequencing Your Kinetic Chain   142

29   Geometry for Kinematic (or Kinetic) Improvements   143

30   Game Day—The Success Point of Your Preparation   147

31   Building Your Tangible and Intangible Teams   149

32   Assessing or Adding to Your Psychological Prep Team   151

33   Clear Those Prep-Psych Issues   152

34   Hire an Invisible Board of Directors—Your Spiritual
Team   152

35   Establish Your Workout Program   154

36   Cycling into a Healing Slumber   166

37   Putting Subtle Energy Crystals in Your Energy Field   173

38   Injury Prevention with Body Awareness   175

39   Psychic Surgery   179

40   Hands-On Healing for Psychic Surgery   180

41   Elemental Healing   180

42   Using Virtual Light to Quicken Healing   182

43 Immediate Protection and Offloading   183

44 Safe Recovery—Motion and Strength   183

45 Reconditioning   184

46 Visualize Your Return   184

47 Go for Freedom   185

48 Programming Through Your Eyes   185

49 Transforming Your Feelings and Awarenesses   191

50 Deep Dreaming   192

51 Do Your Grounding   193

52 Stimulating Your Vagus Nerve   195

53 Align Your Kinetic Chain with the Nadis   197

54 Elemental Boosts   198

55 Freeing Yourself from Others' Energies   210

56 Healing Your Emotions   213

57 Center in Your Spine   215

58 The Young Athlete(s) Inside   251

Workout Tips

1 Chain-Lock Prep Success   155

2 Practice Gamma Gameline   156

3 Seize Authority   156

4 Go with Programming   156

FOREWORD

My name is Ryan Morris, and I am a former professional baseball player with the Cleveland Indians. I was drafted in the fourth round, and my dream was to continue playing as long as possible.

After a shoulder surgery caused an abrupt end to my career, I was determined to get to the root of my shoulder injury and pursued that goal for years. I also decided to become a coach so I could devote a much more personal approach to athletes, something I'd not experienced enough of during my developmental years.

I obtained certifications as a strength coach and biomechanics specialist, and in the course of formulating my coaching career, I ended up taking a very holistic approach to assisting athletes. I call myself the Baseball Mechanic.

During my sessions with athletes, I take an in-depth look at their body alignment, mobility, strength, and soft tissue quality, along with their biomechanics. I know that many one-on-one coaches take this approach, and Cyndi emphasizes this in her book. Her specialty in energy highlights the importance of examining the body, which includes the need to prioritize diet, create strength-building plans, and employ a professional to assess kinetics and mechanics.

In my career, I've come to understand that every athlete is unique in their makeup physically, mentally, emotionally, and spiritually. Therefore, every athlete should have their own custom-built path to success. That path can include various energetic approaches.

Through my experience in my personal work with Cyndi and in working cohesively with her son Gabe, I have discovered an entirely new way to help evaluate my clients. Cyndi has helped me see changes in my athletes' energy like I never had before. I now feel I can read my athletes so much better when it pertains to flaws in their biomechanics. I feel blessed to have worked with Cyndi and Gabe and look forward to my continued work with them.

Ryan Morris

Baseball pitching coach and
former professional MLB pitcher

FOREWORD

It is my distinct pleasure to write this foreword. My first introduction to Cyndi's energy-healing work was well over a decade ago, when I was on a journey of spiritual growth.

I am a practicing cardiologist and have been in the medical field for well over twenty years. Yet there was always a deep inner knowing, a *je ne sais quoi* feeling that there was more to life than the traditional medicine and ethics I had been taught. On my way home from an exhausting day at the hospital, I stopped at a local bookstore and stumbled upon two of Cyndi's books, *The Complete Book of Chakra Healing* and *The Subtle Body Encyclopedia*, while perusing the self-development and healing section.

Perhaps it was an initial energetic attraction to the books as they called to my curious unconscious. I felt that her approach offered the promise of answers to my numerous questions regarding the hows and whys of the affairs of the tangible heart to the metaphysical heart space and its many connections to the human body. Because of that fateful day, I have found the solutions I sought over the years, mainly through figuring out the relationship between energy medicine and the physical body. I have enthusiastically been applying these ideas to my everyday practices, including cardiology and my own physical health.

The well-defined meditations I learned became a part of my daily energetic rituals. I soon discovered that my physical and emotional health improved with the techniques I embraced. Over the years, I continued self-study with more of Cyndi's amazing books, which hold a wealth of knowledge about energy medicine, healing, and wellness. I finally decided one day that I would more directly learn these techniques from Cyndi and apply them with more comprehensive applications. Inspired, I joined her famous Apprenticeship Program and learned from the master teacher herself. What a fantastic experience that was rich with vital information!

My journey did not end there. To this day it continues to grow and evolve, as many such endeavors do. I bridge the worlds of traditional medicine and cardiology and alternative medicine within my evolving practice scope. I regularly discuss these methodologies with my patients, blending the subtle body energetics with the physicalities of the heart space and the body. As an author and inspirational speaker, I also share with audiences and readers worldwide.

As time passed, and as part of my own healing odyssey, I became a CrossFit coach and a competition triathlete. I was blessed to infuse the multitude of Cyndi's energetic wisdom into my life with greater satisfaction and results on all levels of medicine and athleticism. It's exciting how these important concepts can be intertwined with everything, including all levels of sports and athletics. At one level we are all athletes (or ought to be), as movement is a vital part of health and wellness at every level.

To anyone reading this latest beneficial creation by Cyndi, I am enthusiastic about your own personal revelations and transformations that you will encounter. I would invite you to savor them and witness the marvels to be discovered in your athletic journey with the valuable tools found in this book.

Blessings of Love, Light, and Wisdom,

Dr. Nitin Bhatnagar
Holistic heart doctor, cardiologist, author,
life architect, and inspirational speaker

INTRODUCTION

The first time I used an energy technique on my son—in front of other people, anyway—was when he was sixteen.

Gabe and I were in North Carolina at a baseball facility. I had hired two personal trainers to improve Gabe's pitching. As for me? I was just hanging out.

For the most part, throughout all my sports experiences as a mother, I was just a mom in the bleachers. Don't laugh. This is an exclusive club all on its own, made up of lackeys who fill and carry coolers, pack sunscreen and splints, and suffer through natural disasters ranging from summer tornadoes to spring snowstorms. Given that I'm a world-renowned energy healer and intuitive, however, I'd stretched beyond that mom job description hundreds of times.

After all, during the several decades of my career, I've assisted countless athletes—from the everyday variety to the most elite in their fields—in a professional capacity. I've helped a variety of coaches who serve the sports industry as well. Why wouldn't I pass on a few energy tips to my kids and, at the moment, to my youngest son in particular?

However, the informal rules of sports at all levels are clear, and one in particular is sacrosanct: in public there is to be no parental intrusion.

At best, making comments about what you are seeing will get you thrown out of a practice or a game. At worst, your remarks will result in your getting the cold shoulder from your kid for months.

So of course, while sitting on a cold steel bleacher in an unheated facility in wintery Charlotte, I tried to mind my own business. In fact, I was typing away on my laptop, my frigid fingers pecking out yet another book about energy medicine and intuition. But I had a problem: I kept empathically sensing a problem in my son's left arm. I knew he was in pain because my own arm was experiencing sharp shooting sensations, and there was no way my feeble finger movements could be throwing out my arm.

So finally I said something.

"Gabe, is something wrong with your left arm?"

My son looked over at me and blinked. He didn't say anything.

His coaches seemed startled. They obviously hadn't noticed anything, primarily because Gabe is a right-handed pitcher. But I couldn't ignore the ghostly throbbing moving up and down my arm. So I pressed forward. Moms know how to do that.

"It's okay to tell us your left arm aches."

"Yeah," Gabe admitted, holding his left arm with his right hand. "It hurts so bad I can't even lift it." In fact, he couldn't elevate it more than a couple of inches away from his body.

With his trainers peering at us, I conducted my energetic "magic." Within ten minutes Gabe's arm was back to full mobility, with absolutely no residual tenderness.

What did I do? Basically, I used the very same techniques I've employed as a professional energy healer and intuitive for almost 70,000 clients and students over the years. As the author of almost thirty books, I've become quite well known for these concepts and applications, which I've taught in countries including Russia, China, Belize, Costa Rica, Holland, and Peru. After years of working with athletes and coaches "on the sly," however, I'm now going public with the very ideas that I used on Gabe's arm. In a nutshell, what I did for Gabe is called energy medicine.

Absolutely everything is made of energy, from a basketball to the emotions a basketball player experiences during competition. Every challenge afflicting athletes, whether they're aware of it or not, is caused by an energetic problem. And every solution is energetic too. In fact—again, whether they know it or not—sports coaches, from the volunteer Little League parent to the specialist trainer, are constantly instructing those under their care in energetics, with *energy* defined simply as information that vibrates.

The other part of the equation, *medicine*, is anything that creates more ease. I didn't do anything obvious to loosen up Gabe's arm; I delivered *subtle* rather than physical energies.

As I'll further explain in this book, there are two basic types of energy. One side of the coin is physical energy. We focus on this type of energy in sports all the time, such as when gauging pounds lifted, miles run, mechanical accuracy, macro- and micronutrients, and the like. Physical fixes and tools absolutely matter. They are a vital part of the athletic equation, whether you're a hiker or a pro football player. I'll talk about some of these physical factors in this book.

However, 99.999 percent of what appears in our everyday reality is actually made of invisible energy, the stuff I call "subtle energy." For that reason, this book is going to teach you everything you need to know as an athlete—or a coach—about subtle energy and sports performance. Because I'm going to give you working tools from the energy medicine kit bag, I'll usually call this approach "energy work" instead of "energy medicine." It does take work, as you'll see, but it's so productive.

I know that this approach works in sports because I've seen it work again and again. I've used the techniques in this book to help an injured football player's medial collateral ligament (MCL) heal in half the average recovery time. With my support, a washed-out downhill skier regained passion and confidence and started winning competitions again. I was thrilled when a young high school softball player boosted her abilities enough to earn a scholarship to college, and I assisted a seventy-five-year-old woman in figuring out and sticking to a training program to prepare for a spiritual quest in Spain. In fact, I once sent subtle energies into the broken hand of a volleyball player in front of a small group. We all gasped as the golf ball–sized swelling disappeared in front of our eyes.

The concepts of energetic work and subtle energy aren't totally alien to the world of sports. Maybe you've heard of or perhaps used some of the most basic energy medicine techniques such as hypnotherapy, which is guided hypnosis; Reiki, the delivery of universal healing energies; acupuncture, the use of needles to stimulate *chi*, or life energy; and even prayer, which involves requesting assistance from a higher power. Perhaps you're even aware of vibrational remedies, including tools such as flower essences, crystals, and more.

There are so many other effective methods, though, and I want you to know the best of the best of them, whether you're an everyday athlete, an elite one, or a coach. And guess what? As a parent, you're also a coach.

Are you ready for this journey? Here is a brief map of what you'll discover in the two parts of this book. In a nutshell, part 1 (chapters 1 through 4) teaches you about energy and sports and presents your most important energy techniques. Then in part 2 (chapters 5 through 11), I cover the major areas of sports interest.

Following are more details.

Chapter 1: Important terms and science. Let's start this outing on the same field. After defining terms like "athlete," "coach," and "performance," we'll examine the main areas of interest we'll be covering in this book such as performance, injury prevention and care, and exactly why energetic concepts and tools can make such a huge difference in sports.

Chapter 2: Energy as causal. Energy is the root cause of all sports problems, but it can also provide all the needed antidotes. We'll cover the lengthy list of the types of energies that create "blocks," or challenges, for the athlete.

3

Chapter 3: The energy system. Here you will learn all about the subtle energetic system and how it interrelates with your mind and body. Chakras, anyone? How about auric fields, meridians, and frequencies? They are all here.

Chapter 4: Get-set techniques. Time to pick up the ball/bat/racket/whistle (you get it). The concepts and techniques in this chapter will prep you for ever-improving performance.

Chapter 5: Failure and success. Short and sweet, let's examine the three p's of performance failure and the three p's of success.

Chapter 6: Mechanics. No matter the game, mechanics are key. How do you accomplish great mechanics without sliding into perfectionism? We'll look at famous greats who did it their own way and provide tools and tips for doing the same.

Chapter 7: Preparation. Every game starts with preparation, and there are powerful energetic and vibrational keys that will help you create and follow through on your prep.

Chapter 8: Injuries. It happens to everyone. The human body is prone to injury. What energetic ideas and techniques can assist with injury prevention, care, and recovery? You will learn those here.

Chapter 9: Performance. It's game day, whatever that means to you! What tricks of the subtle trade can get you through the pre-performance jitters and any game mishaps? How do you handle the negativity of foes, including your own inner saboteur? I'll even give a few tips for specific sports.

Chapter 10: The winding road. There will be ups and downs. It's vital to establish and then return to your plumb line for stability. Help yourself—or the athlete in your life—maintain equilibrium and, if necessary, pull out of a downward spiral.

Chapter 11: For coaches. In a way, almost everyone around an athlete is a coach. That includes parents, volunteer and paid referees, trainers, and medical professionals. You might even be an athlete who helps other athletes. How do you help yourself while doing that work? How can you keep yourself up when the athlete goes up and down? This chapter also gives specifics about how to adapt this book's techniques to assist a young person. We'll also examine the "inner children" within you. We all have them: echoes of your younger selves who hold trauma as well as talent.

As you can see, there is a lot of information on the energetics of sports between these covers that you won't find anywhere else. No matter what else you learn, this book will help you get to the most important place of all: the energetic self inside you. Take away what you see and you get to the subtle—the spirit, both of yourself and sports.

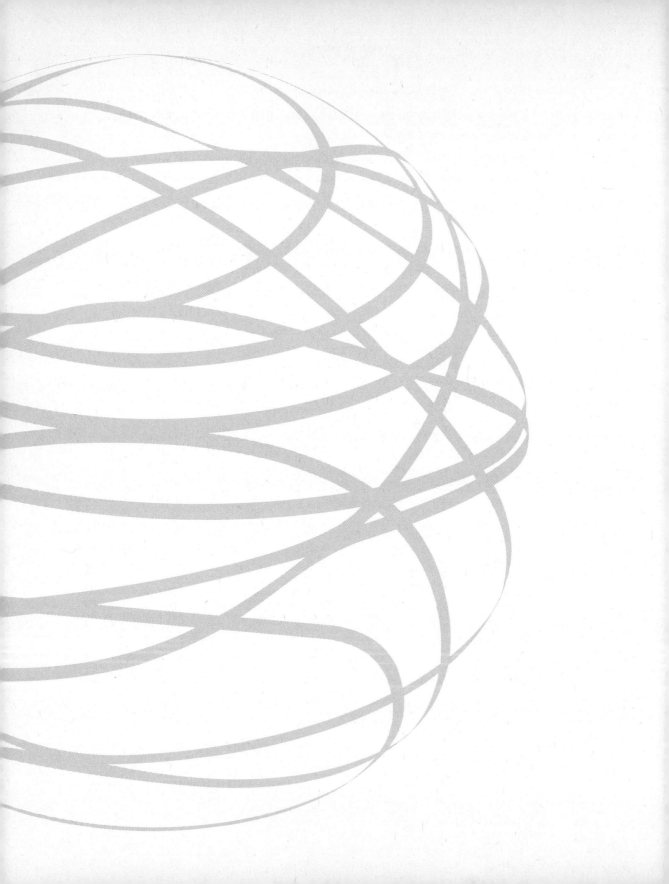

PART 1

Get Ready and Set!

There isn't a game in the world that can be played without first laying the groundwork. Nor is there a coach who can coach decently without having a sense of what they need to accomplish.

The four chapters in part 1 are all about preparing you to become the best athlete or coach you can be. A lot of books say they'll do that, but this one is different because chances are, most of this information will be brand-new for you. Here I will cover the basics of energetics so you will understand these important principles and why energy work is so beneficial for the sports world. I'll also introduce you to subtle energy anatomy. It's your "partner in crime"—and in winning solutions—to physical energy anatomy, and it's much more powerful!

This first part of the book is like a pep rally for where we're going. It's chock-full of the fundamental energy techniques and vibrational remedies you need to know to achieve real performance highs.

Get ready ... get set ... *here we go!*

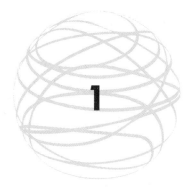

1

How Energetics Boosts Sports of All Sorts

When the mind is controlled and spirit
aligned with purpose, the body is capable
of so much more than we realize.
—Rich Roll, endurance athlete, in *Finding Ultra*

My client was crying. Trained in dance since age seven, she had repeatedly competed for a lead part in her jazz-dance specialty. She had been passed over just as frequently.

During one of our first sessions, we got to the bottom of the issue. The problem wasn't the result of mechanics, injury, or a downward spiral. Mental stress was a factor. Who in her situation wouldn't become depressed and self-questioning? But the core issue wasn't one that a typical sports therapist or trainer would have uncovered.

It's called an "energy marker," and you'll learn all about it in chapter 4. Basically, there are forms of invisible energies that, once attached to a person, compel mistreatment by other people. That's right! Think of an energy marker as a great big sticky note pasted on the body. Written on it are words that face the outside world. People susceptible to that message, because of their own inner programming, "read" the note and respond in kind.

In the case of my dancer client, the note insisted, "Don't let this person succeed."

I perceived this energy marker intuitively. In fact, I could read it in my mind's eye. Intuition is one of the most important tools you'll employ to wield the powerful energetic techniques in this book, and I'll help you activate and employ your own intuitive gifts, also in chapter 4. You'll learn to pay attention to your intuition—because it's always right.

As my dancer client put it, "Yes! I've always felt like there was a bad luck sign on me. How can I get it off?"

We did the deep-dive to discover that a jealous sister had inadvertently pinned this sign on her. Of course, the sister hadn't meant to create harm, but damage had been done; most of what we do to others, and they do to us, is done subconsciously. Upon reflection, my client realized that the problem didn't occur only in sports; she hadn't climbed to the top of any ladder. Once a strong candidate for a scholarship, she'd just missed making the cut. If interviewed for a media outlet, her insights never made it to the public.

As you'll discover, once you locate the subtle challenge, you can use any number of easy subtle energy tools to undo much of the damage—and then leap higher than ever. That's what happened with my client. After a few sessions, she was able to release that negative subtle marker. And within a few weeks after that, she landed her first lead part.

And here's what I want you to understand about that: it's not magic. It's energy.

Sports Are a Matter of Energy

I know you've experienced the difference between feeling energized and not. When you're highly energized, you can push, persevere, and play. But when your energy is low? You're off, limited, and lacking in motivation. Workouts feel like they take a really *l-o-n-g* time, as does just about anything you do for your sport.

At that point, you want a miracle.

This reminds me of the time Gabe asked me to go outside and play with him. I told him I was too tired.

"Why don't you just put in a new battery?" he suggested. "It sounds like your old one is all worn out."

Energy work doesn't guarantee the exact same outcome as putting in a spanking new battery, but it does connect you to an endless source of energy. From there, you can pull in what you need so you can do what must be done. To put this concept to work, you have to begin with an understanding of energy.

As I expressed in the introduction, energy is simply information that vibrates. So what does this mean in general, but also when applied to sports?

Information is the influence that tells energy how to materialize. In other words, it's data. It tells that "something" to be a lacrosse stick rather than a bumper sticker. This important data isn't found only inside of an object; it also lies outside of it.

Let's take a baseball. There is a code that makes it a ball with a white surface laced with seams. When a pitcher picks it up and throws? *Whomp!* The pitcher's intention is going to change that ball. Though you might not notice it, the surface area will be different post-pitch and certainly post-hit.

Want another example of external influences? Take the rules used by a referee in football. Those rules are data, and they will determine whether a football caught beyond the line of scrimmage will be live or not. Your game, whatever it is, can be made or broken by external information.

The other part of our energy formula is vibration. There are many ways to define vibration. At the most basic level, vibration is movement. In fact, absolutely everything is constantly moving. That includes objects, people, and even the invisible subcomponents of what appears to be really solid. That's right: molecules, atoms, and subatomic quanta—the smallest known units of reality—are all in constant motion.

When something is moving, it is going back and forth or maybe up and down and perhaps in every direction at once. Technically, these oscillations are occurring at various frequencies, a frequency being the number of occurrences of an event that repeat during a certain time period. You're going to discover that your ability to perform during a competition or even succeed at a workout program is going to come down to frequencies. But until I talk about that more in chapter 3, ruminate on how important vibration is to your sports abilities.

Let's return to our baseball. If you're a baseball pitcher, the difference between a hittable and non-hittable pitch often comes down to vibration. After all, the amount of spin on a pitch changes its trajectory. Is that throw going to barely miss home plate or might it cross over "just so"? The wibble-wobble that determines the ump's call of "ball" or "strike" is vibratory.

And in baseball, even the vibration of the bat is all-important. *Smack!* Bat hits ball—and sets off a vibration. Want to hit a pitch out of the park? That incoming pitch has to be spinning or vibrating really fast or it won't carry enough power to get that hit ball up and out. In fact, batters unconsciously clue in to the best way to hit that ball based on vibratory clues like the sound made upon contact and the perceived route of the incoming ball. These vibratory issues are equally true in cricket, golf, tennis, hockey, hurling, softball, and other sports.[1]

What's the bad news/good news implication of our definition of energy for the athlete or the coach?

- ▸ The causes of all sports-related problems are energetic. After all, everything is made of energy, so that's a logical conclusion. (somewhat bad news)

- ▸ The solutions for all sports-related issues are also energetic. (good news)

- ▸ To create an antidote for an athletic challenge, you can alter either information or vibration or both. (good news)

- ▸ To complicate matters, however, there are two different types of energy, as I've already been telling you. (somewhat bad news, as this fact can complicate your approach)

- ▸ However, this means that you have a lot of choices for how to transform a problem into an incredible opportunity. (good news)

You'll be able to turn the bad news—or somewhat bad news—into good news with a little more understanding of our two types of energy.

The Two Types of Energy and What They Mean for the Athlete

I've already said that there are both physical and subtle forms of energy. What does this distinction mean in the world of sports?

We can't be successful at a sport without considering physical energies. In fact, the most common definition of energy is "the ability to perform work." The very definition of the word *athlete*, a person who is good at sports and other forms of physical exercise, means that to perform, you have to focus on improving your relationship with the physical energies inside and outside of yourself. You have to work out, wear appropriate clothing, eat healthy foods, get enough sleep, and do an awful lot of push-ups. Your age or your sport doesn't matter; physical actions are necessary to create improvement.

---

1 Russell, "Acoustics and Vibration."

The easiest way to arrive at a precise understanding of physical energies and their relation to the world of sports is to think of the equipment you need. If you're a badminton player, at the top of the list is a badminton racket. You know it's made of physical energy because you can see, touch, and even smell it. (Not that you usually go around doing that, but …) Heck, you can even taste the racket, if you want to! When the racket is whizzing through the air, you can also hear it. All five of your normal senses key you in to physical energies.

Besides being measurable through our regular senses, physical energies are also pretty obvious to others. After all, you aren't the only one who can tell that's a badminton racket sitting there.

As an athlete, you have to be constantly concerned about physical energies. If the badminton racket is broken or improperly strung, that's going to negatively affect your performance. If it's in tip-top shape and you're not doing so well, you'd better look at yourself.

Sports coaches nearly always focus on the importance of physical energies and the tools used to work with them. A sports coach is someone who supports an athlete in reaching their potential. Athletes need lots of different types of sports coaches to boost them in seeking to achieve their goals. The group often includes parents, volunteer coaches or trainers, paid or unpaid mentors, sports psychologists, and bloggers and other sports authorities, but it also includes an entourage of assistants like physical therapists and physicians. Plus, if you're an athlete, I recommend that you think of yourself as one of your own coaches! After all, you spend an awful lot of time helping yourself along, don't you?

The truth is, an athlete requires much more than physical assists. This is why so many athletes and coaches are already grasping for ways to assess and command subtle energies, whether they know it or not. Think of it: when you're focused on your mental game, emotional responses, reactions to negativity, or ways to calm yourself when you're freaked, you're actually working with subtle energies. You're also trying to tap into a nearly boundless sea of power that can assist you with every part of your sport or aid someone else in doing the same.

Unfortunately, it's harder to define subtle energies than physical ones, even though the subtle ones make up more than 99 percent of all energy. That's because they aren't easily measurable. Also called psychic, intuitive, bioenergetic, and quantum energies, they are, however, the elusive but all-powerful keys to the universe, including the world of athletics.

The most accurate way to explain subtle energies is through the lens of quantum physics. This area is the study of quanta, which are subatomic—or very tiny—fields of energy. These aren't just any old energies. In fact, they love to color outside the lines of 3D reality, as I'll share next.

Quanta, or subtle energies:

- *only become really "here" or "real" when they are observed.* This means that until you really swing at, kick, lob, wallop, or do whatever it is you do to the ball or whatever tool you use in your sport, anything is possible. And that means the more time or focus you expend practicing what you want to accomplish, the easier it becomes to get those quanta to do what you want.

- *can jump from one state to another.* From a physics perspective, they operate like waves—which ripple across time and space—as well as particles, which are fixed. For the athlete or the coach supporting them, this means that no matter how stuck the situation is, you can shift it. Have an injury? Came in last place? Challenged in your training? Unable to stay on the best diet? That doesn't need to be the case forever!

- *go wherever the heck they want—when they aren't being watched.* Okay, we just said that quanta aren't totally present until they are being observed. (Sort of like toddlers in a room who won't sit until the teacher insists.) A cool consequence of this fact is that when no one is watching—when you take your mind off the ball—those quanta can get really creative. They can move around and then presto: you can potentially call them into a very different place. Why not let your quanta solve a problem while you ignore it? Why not give permission for your roving quanta to visit a place that holds much-needed healing energy while you place your mind elsewhere?

- *obey something strange called the Uncertainty Principle.* This theory says that we can't know both the location and the movement of a quantum at the same time. (Now, stay with me. This is a complicated but really big deal.) If that's true, our dreams must obey natural law, and come true in a relatively slow way. But ... scientists figured out that you *can* determine the position and momentum of a quantum if it is going faster than the speed of light.[2]

Do you know what can go faster than the speed of light? Information with no mass, or weight. *Sort of like your unbridled but directed desires.*

Yes, this is cool. It means that your wishes really can come true because they can move super fast and get you beyond your current performance.

In chapter 4 I'm going to give you a specific exercise to help you send ideas into the universe on a specific type of energy called scalar waves that move information faster than the speed of light. I also call these waves "Healing Streams of Grace" because I believe that grace—or love in motion—is made up of these waves. Using this particular wave of energy, you can learn how to make changes to how your history, current reality, and even future affect you. Such alterations can actually make real-life adjustments to anything from your mechanics to the sites of injuries. For instance, what if your mechanics don't need to be negatively affected by a long-ago injury, even if the injury means you won't fully return to the level of performance you once had?

▸ *always spin or rotate around an axis.* Yes, even though they are very tiny and seemingly nonsequential, quanta still organize around a center point. That is good news for the athlete because you'll discover that if you are centered in your axis, such as your spine, you can control important mechanical constructs and even your actual speed. You can also achieve the mental equilibrium necessary to enter *flow*: the ability to naturally and instinctively move and shift with events. I believe you'll love exercise 38, which enables you to obtain this exact state.

▸ *once connected, remain connected and continue to affect each other.* That's right. If two quanta—or people or objects—get to know each other, even just by passing each other on a ball field or on a track, they remain linked. That is called "quantum entanglement." What affects one can influence the other.

---

2   Dale, *Advanced Chakra Healing*, 71–72.

Now we're back to the bad news/good news.

Bad news: If you lost to a team before, you are more inclined to do so again. You'll have channels open to take in the chiding or negativity.

Good news: If someone you know is silently supporting you, like a mom in the bleachers or even a friend halfway around the world who is thinking about you, their positivity can boost your performance.

In the end, you've actually heard this quantum stuff before, most likely in terms such as the power of positive thinking. In a nutshell, this says "become what you think you can become." But that concept only works once you've truly mastered your comprehension and the direction of the subtle energies that affect your athleticism.

Want more proof? From the non-sporty world, consider Mahendra Kumar Trivedi, known as Trivedi or Guruji.

In 1995 Guruji began to change physical reality by administering simple blessings. For a few minutes at a time, he would simply focus on a situation he wanted to change in a positive way. Studies have shown that his blessings accomplished concrete feats. For instance, they increased seed germination and survival rates among blessed plants to 99.5 percent, compared to 60 to 65 percent in control crops,[3] and even boosted control yields in a chickpea plot 350 percent over control yields.[4]

What is a blessing but a prayer, an intention, a focused way to shift subtle energies? I've personally seen athletes who have shifted their abilities to an incredible degree with a simple grasp of this idea.

James is a young British man I worked with who was attending a preparatory school on the East Coast of the United States. James loved tennis. In fact, he lived and breathed for tennis and was sure that his life would be meaningless unless he could become a professional tennis player. His mother asked me to work with him to help him get better at tennis because he was at best a Division III tennis player.

In America, colleges and universities with sports programs are labeled by divisions. Divisions are based on the size of the school, the level of competition, and the funding of the athletic program. Division I schools are well funded and can award fairly sizeable scholar-

---

3 Vidyapeeth and Krishi, "Alphonso Mango."
4 Bohra, "Response of Mustard and Chickpea."

ships. Division II schools pass out much smaller scholarships, and Division III schools don't award any monies. In general, the most elite players—those with the best chances of going pro—usually attend Division I schools, although it's not impossible for athletes to stretch into success through any division.

In terms of my young client, James didn't stand much of a chance of attending a school with a decent tennis standing, much less going pro.

We worked together five times. I used the basic techniques you'll learn in chapter 4. By the end of that term, he was being recruited by Division I and Division II schools. Not only that, but his grades had also raised a full level, and he felt confident enough to gain his first-ever girlfriend. What made the most difference? His self-esteem grew once he understood that he was in charge of his own subtle energies. With that idea uppermost, he started to make small changes that resulted in big rewards.

What is interesting, however, is that in the end he accepted an offer to a Division II school. Over the course of the semester, his goals had changed. He decided he wanted to be a professional engineer, not a tennis player, although he wanted to continue playing tennis for fun. I don't consider him an athletic failure; rather, this young man transformed into more of his true self. In other words, he become more conscious.

The Relationship Between Physical and Subtle Energies—and Consciousness

One of the central concepts the energized athlete has to grasp is that physical and subtle energies flow into each other. Quite simply, one type of energy converts into the other, with the most solid of physical energies on one side of a continuum and the most far-out, wild, hardly-even-anywhere subtle energies on the other. What's in between? The subtle energy anatomy—and what powers the transition of energies: your consciousness.

The subtle energy anatomy, which we'll outline thoroughly in chapter 3, consists of subtle organs, fields, and channels. By the way, the same could be said of your physical anatomy—except the organs, fields, and channels are physical, not subtle. These three aspects of the anatomy are going to be vital to comprehend as you'll interact with them to make your athletic dreams come true.

The main subtle organs (or centers) you'll be putting to work through this book are your chakras. They are comparable to your physical organs, like your heart or liver, but ever so much more powerful in that you can create change in the physical body via your chakras.

We'll work with twelve chakras, some of which are anchored inside the body and some outside. Through your chakras, you can change physical to subtle energies (and vice versa) and actually steer your subtle energies. For you coaches out there, you can also assist your athletes in doing the same.

Your auric fields are layers of light and sound (called auric layers) that emanate from your chakras to encompass your physical self. The layers basically manage the you outside of you. Are you vulnerable to others' negativity? Are there certain environments that make you feel at a disadvantage? Clearing these types of susceptibilities and enhancing your strong and focused self are a matter of working with these fields.

Finally, we come to the existence of subtle energy channels. There are two types, as we'll further explore: the meridians and the nadis. They operate a lot like the physical channels flowing through your body, including the lymph and blood vessels, except they carry both subtle and physical energies throughout your system. Want to manage your nerves, digestion, feelings, and more? Learn how to better administer your subtle energy channels by using the techniques in this book.

Even this brief description of your subtle anatomy begs a greater question: How exactly are you going to steer subtle energies, no matter how much knowledge you gain of your invisible self? The answer is by using your consciousness.

At the most basic level, consciousness is awareness. To be conscious implies that you are aware of yourself and the outside world. It infers that you comprehend your impact on the environment and the environment's on you. However, you can be perceptive without being empowered.

To be a great athlete or coach, you have to cultivate empowered consciousness. You need to be certain of what occurs inside and outside of the self or other, be guided by a higher goal or ethic, and know what to do about what isn't working.

Our main tool for consciousness in sports development is intuition. Intuition is your ability to receive, interpret, shape, create, and send subtle energies, or the invisible information that vibrates. After all, we respond to the world based on the information we bring in and what we think it means. The world will also treat us the way we subtly insist it does.

Think about a goalie. The puck slices through the air toward the net—and the goalie blocks it! To whom should she now direct the puck? Tuned in to her intuition, the goalie senses that Skater A is distracted and not ready to go. Skater B, on the other hand, even though not positioned as well, seems on the ball—or puck, that is. There goes the puck.

This goalie has used her intuition to determine the meaning of the subtle energies coming into her system and to respond accordingly.

Our goalie can also determine how Skater B might respond to this power position. Remember that less than 1 percent of an object is physical. How might the goalie impact Skater B by sending a "you can do it" message? Especially if the other possibility is "you're going to blow this"? Some scientists actually think that information is the basis of the universe. If you don't like what exists, break apart the information formula and build it up again using new data.[5]

Other scientists, however, theorize that vibration is king—or queen. It's all about resonance, or matching vibrations, which create the patterns that make up 3D reality.[6] Change the vibration—or speed, spin, or the like—and you impact the outcome. No matter your preference for information or vibration or both, you have to become more conscious of what's happening with subtle energy if you want to bring about better outcomes.

Scientific Theories of Energetic Transformation

Let me start this section by letting you know that reading it is optional. Some people are really into the science of how stuff works; some aren't. I've written this section for those who want a deeper understanding of the science of energetic transformation—or how you make a difference by changing subtle energies. So if it's not that interesting to you, you have a pass. Just skip ahead! I'll meet you at the Energetics in Sports section further along.

But if you want to move forward, I am going to tie the science—and one researcher and his research in particular—to athletics. Allow me to introduce you to a man whose research reveals the incredible power of subtle energies and the science behind them as forces for change. Meet Royal Raymond Rife, a scientist, inventor, and engineer back in the 1930s.

I'll paint a picture of him for you. He's a thin, dark-haired, intense man clothed in a white coat. He's in his laboratory, and he's really excited to show you what he's done.

Rife has invented a microscope so powerful that it enables him to see the tiniest of pathogens, which can't be perceived using the other microscopes of this time. His invention is called the Rife Universal Microscope. Magnifying 60,000 times, it uses monochromatic light to make the microbes appear fluorescent. Using this unique process, Rife differentiates

5 Perry, "The Basis of the Universe."
6 Hunt, "The Hippies Were Right."

various microbes based on the colors refracted off them. Certain microbes show as one specific color, and others appear as different colors.

Rife knows everything that exists vibrates at its own particular frequency. His research has revealed three radical outcomes, which I'm not only going to describe but link to athletic success.

> *1: The effects and impacts of a microbe can depend on its environment.* Through his research, Rife has discovered a virus that causes cancer in breast tissue. He's also found out that the terrain (or environment) of the breast determines the form and lethality of the virus.
>
> This *theory of pleomorphism* is critical for the athlete. It explains why you can skillfully pitch/run/catch/think/push/pull/skate/hit/lob or do whatever you do in your sport in certain environments—or around specific people—but not do very well in or near others. How you perform is at least partially a matter of the negativity and positivity of the ecosystem around you, including the attitudes and opinions of others.
>
> *2: Everything resonates at its own optimum frequency.* This means that differing frequencies can either support or destroy something else that has frequencies.
>
> For instance, Rife has found that if he figures out the frequency of a cancer virus, he can then destroy that virus with a "mortality frequency" of the same nature. In fact, after determining the frequency of a cancer virus, he then fires at it with a radio wave (packaged in a specific way) of a comparable frequency. The microbe is eliminated. Using this method, he heals cancer in fourteen of sixteen people within seventy days during a human trial in 1934. The other two individuals are pronounced cured in another three weeks.[7]
>
> Studies since Rife's have shown that an array of frequencies are able to initiate healing in individuals, especially when delivered as sound. A review of four hundred published studies underscores the evidence that music can create actual health benefits. For instance, sound-based vibration has also decreased pain and arthritis and resulted in increased blood circulation and lower blood pressure.[8]

7   Sadeghi and Sami, "Forgotten Genius."
8   Wei, "The Healing Power of Sound."

This theory of resonance shows that, if you are dedicated, you can empower yourself (or coach another) to become free of illness, injuries, and even negative beliefs. You can also administer subtle energies, in the form of frequencies, to enhance anything from attitude to activity. Overall, becoming an expert at subtle (invisible) frequencies and vibrations is key to many aspects of your performance.

3: *Frequencies determine positive, neutral, or negative impacts.* Additional studies by Rife reveal that different frequencies, when aimed at microbes, can change them from one type of microbe into another type altogether. This endeavor can also alter a lethal microbe and make it nonlethal, and vice versa.[9]

This theory of transformation means that nothing is ever stuck at "bad." At the very least, you can shift negative to neutral—and maybe even into positive! And that's the name of the game.

Let's say you become conscious of being able to transform energies. What might be the sports benefits?

Energetics in Sports: The Stages Leading to Great Performance

As we've been discussing, the rules of energy mean that when you make a change in the subtle universe, exponential effects show up in the physical world. They also mean that when you focus on the physical while embracing the subtle energies also involved, every action you take is bolstered.

In sports, the single most important goal is improvement in performance: the accomplishment of carrying out a task or function. But there are steps and stages that lead to performance, all of which can be nurtured with dedicated consciousness and energetics. Let's take a look at these stages, which mirror the chapters in part 2, and some real people who accomplished great tasks within them.

Mechanics

We don't need perfect mechanics to perform well in our sport, but we must have good enough mechanics to do the job. This often involves figuring out how to adapt mechanics,

---

9   Dale, *Llewellyn's Complete Book of Chakras*, 375.

or proper body sequencing, of our sport function to our own body. This can be best done using subtle techniques, either solo or in conjunction with making physical changes.

EXAMPLE: Brian was a professional ice skater who continually struggled to carry off a double axel. Sometimes he could and sometimes he couldn't, and the inconsistency was causing stress in his traveling company. His skating coach said it was a mechanical or sequencing issue.

An axel is a tough trick. It requires the ability to take off on the forward edge of a skate and requires an extra half-turn for completion. Together, Brian and I figured out that he was twisting his spine when in the air. No matter how often he tried to make manual improvements, they didn't hold. So we dug underneath, into the subtleties.

During a regression, which is a process for returning to and remembering the past, Brian remembered being tossed off a cliff during a past life. He had fallen to his death. That terror, which had stuck in his soul, had downloaded into his current body and was still stuck there. Every time he twisted in a certain way, the trauma came up again—hence, his inability to hold his spine the right way during an axel jump.

Yes, you see that I believe in past lives. I'll address this concept more in chapter 2, but just bear with me for right now.

In order to change his posturing, Brian processed the old emotions. He also supported the release of the fear with flower essences: vibrational remedies that helped him integrate a change in body, mind, and soul. You'll learn about these in chapter 4! After a few more months of practicing the axel while dealing with the old emotions, Brian was able to consistently pull off the move. His spine still didn't hold his posture perfectly, but it didn't throw him off either. As you'll learn, perfect isn't necessary, not when your subtle energies are working for you.

Preparation

Even if you're "merely" a weekend warrior, you still have to get in shape to perform. No matter your sport or your level of development, performance usually includes creating and implementing a workout plan, which often entails activities like stretching, strength building, lifting, and increasing agility; adherence to a spot-on nutritional program; mental and emotional balancing; and more.

EXAMPLE: Estrella is the English name of a Chinese woman who practiced tai chi on the streets with her friends every morning. I worked with her long distance over Zoom once a month for several months.

For the past year, she'd felt achy after her morning exercises. Quite simply, she wasn't preparing the way she used to.

Many athletes spend most of their time in preparation. But Estrella was simply rolling out of bed and heading to the park. She didn't eat well, stretch out, or even wear weather-appropriate clothes. Since she had done all those things before, the question was, what had blocked her devotion to preparation?

Estrella shared that the year before, her mother had moved in with her. Then came the nagging. No matter what, Estrella simply wasn't perfect enough for her mother. The emotional negativity was triggering Estrella's issues from childhood, and she began avoiding everything important in her life. We eventually sussed out that the real issue was that in childhood Estrella had taken on her mother's negative feelings and self-judgments. As you'll learn in the next chapter, others' subtle energies actually can take up room in your own body. You can't process energies that aren't your own, so Estrella was depressed with somebody else's feelings.

Together, we worked on cleansing these energies using the techniques in this book. Her attitude and physical energy improved dramatically, and she actually become the leader of her tai chi group.

Injury Prevention, Care, and Recovery

Injuries occur for all athletes. Some are serious, some not, but they are a very real part of sports. Energetics is an extraordinarily important tool for preventing injuries and caring for those that do occur.

EXAMPLE: A few years ago, I worked with a high-end basketball player who had broken his ankle; foot and ankle injuries are among the chief injuries of basketball. When first talking with Ernie, I discovered that he had actually rolled that same ankle many times but had never paid attention. In fact, he usually ignored most of his injuries. Then, *wonk!* During one game, there went the ankle.

My client knew that he was out for the season, but he wanted to get up and moving again quicker than the physical therapists and other coaching crew thought acceptable. My main goal was to help him heal while preventing further damage. I wasn't so sure about him making his way back as quickly as he wanted to, but I was willing to see what we could do.

We first tracked Ernie's pattern of ignoring his aches and pains. He had been raised in a family that pretty much disregarded him. All he had was basketball, but even there, his family never showed up for his games. No one seemed to care what he was going through, so why should he, even if it hurt?

We worked through the chakra relating to relationships. By doing so, Ernie eventually began to perceive that not only did he love the game with his whole heart, but he needed to love himself with the same intensity. Once he accepted this fact, the subtle energies we delivered into his ankle with hands-on techniques, which you'll learn in this book, actually took hold. He healed three weeks quicker than expected, and though he didn't return for the season, he was a smashing success for the next one.

Game Day

"Game day" isn't always the day of an actual game. All athletes have success benchmarks, however, whether they are imposed from the inside or the outside. Energetics can be crucial to feeling good and doing great on game day, whatever game day means to you.

EXAMPLE: One of my own game day stories occurred a few years ago when I decided to walk part of the Camino de Santiago from Portugal to Santiago de Compostela, Spain. The Camino is a set of paths that has been walked by pilgrims for hundreds of years. My friends and I wanted to earn a certificate that involved completing 100 kilometers of tracked walking, so we spent months preparing. In addition, we first walked about 60 kilometers in Lisbon to get our walking legs on.

Perhaps you would not find this type of trip strenuous. It was for us, however, as the odyssey included terrains as diverse as mountain peaks and riverbeds and weather including heat, cold, and rain.

This game day was long: ten days. It was physically taxing, but I found the emotional challenges were equally hard. Five women on a walk? Come on. It's like the theme of that song: *feelings, nothing more than feelings.*

How did I cope? Daily, I cleansed my chakras and pulled up energy from the earth to keep myself moving forward. I fortified my energetic boundaries—the fields around the body—so I didn't take on or react to others' emotions or challenges. And I used deep breathing exercises, such as the one I'll share at the end of this chapter. I also stayed in touch with my goal and my purpose, and used my intuition to get input from my spiritual guides. Yup: in this book, you'll learn that we have invisible yet active spiritual guides who can be of great help on game day and at any other time.

And by the way, who says you are ever too old for a game day?

The Ups and Downs

If there is anything consistent about athletes, it's that we'll be inconsistent. Our physical prowess will rise and fall, as will our emotions. Fortunately, energetics can even out the roller coasters.

EXAMPLE: Janie was an exceptionally talented volleyball player who failed to take advantage of a setup during an important game. Her spike should have ended the game—but she missed the ball altogether. Her self-confidence spiraled, and she began failing other routine plays, even missing most of her serves.

I call this the "downward spiral." We let ourselves down once, and our performance begins to fall. It can be really hard to snatch ourselves out of this vortex-like plunge.

As you'll learn in chapter 10, once our subtle energies start moving downward, they often keep doing so. She began using exercise 52 to deliberately shift her energy on the court—and it worked. Within a few weeks, she was back to normal. You'll get lots of other ideas for prepping for—and performing during—game day in chapter 9.

Coaching Self and Others

If you're an athlete, you need to be your own coach. When you're standing on that lonely mound, moving across the track and field solo, or pulling back the bow for the arrow, that moment is all on you.

Likewise, if you're one of the many different types of coaches supporting an athlete, there is a lot resting on your shoulders. The techniques in this book can be culled to assist you in your endeavors, but you might also need to use some of them for yourself.

EXAMPLE: Scott was a dad in the baseball bleachers, but he didn't feel good about that role as he had absolutely no knowledge of baseball. His young son kept striking out, and he felt like it was partially his fault. Scott couldn't even show him how to hold a bat, and since the coaches didn't have extra time—and he didn't have extra money to hire independent coaches—he just kept feeling worse and worse.

Our first task was to boost Scott's confidence. We dug into some deep sorrows that lingered between him and his own father. The latter had abandoned him at every turn, so of course Scott was especially hard on himself. It took a while to convince him that he wasn't the same as his father—he just didn't understand baseball, that's all. Scott became willing to sort of be his own coach by feeling better about himself. At this point, I asked Scott to start watching baseball games with his son.

Together, they began to study mechanics and plays. Scott also integrated several of the techniques from this book into his son's practice by using the information covered in chapter 3 in relationship to frequencies (see figure 4) and many of the exercises from chapter 4. Yup, he could coach from the bleachers—without saying a thing! His son began to truly enjoy the game and was frequently played.

The Young Athlete

There are special considerations for applying these techniques to our youth, and one of them is to consider the child within.

Yes, inside each athlete, and often each coach, is the young self who has had good and bad experiences with sports. Energetics can be especially beneficial for healing sports wounds and accentuating innate talents and dreams.

EXAMPLE: When I was young, I was traumatized by years spent being forced to play softball in a church youth group. I hated it. I was scared of the ball. I hated running. I couldn't stand competition. I don't think I ever hit the ball. In left field, where I was constantly stuck, I hung back as far as possible, hoping a ball wouldn't come my way.

When Gabe, my youngest, really took to the game, I knew I had to do some deep healing. So I did! I diligently used the techniques that I provide in this book to help my inner child face her fears and embarrassment. As my own healer, I then encouraged her to not only learn the game, but to like it. I now know way too much about baseball, but I love it!

As you can see, change is possible when we understand it's all about energy. We'll further explore the pluses and minuses of energy in the next chapter.

EXERCISE 1: THE FOUR-SIX BREATH

In order to summon our best subtle and physical energies, it's helpful to know how to breathe appropriately. This exercise will teach you a simple breathing technique you can use during any sports endeavor to create calm, summon your inner power, and draw on the unlimited subtle energies of the universe—and it's easy.

This breath technique should be done through the mouth.

Breathe in deeply to the count of four. Then hold your breath at the top of your lungs for a second. Up here, you fill with your potential.

Now exhale for six seconds. Pause at the bottom of the exhalation for a second. Deep inside of you is what scientists call the void, or an endless sea of positive energy. After connecting with this space, relax and inhale for four seconds again.

You can perform this exercise for up to ten cycles and return to your normal breathing when you're done.

When you're finished with the cycles, relax.

———————————

Everything is made of energy, although there are physical (tangible) and subtle (intangible or quantum) forms of energy. We can convert one into another and, by doing so, release athletic problems and open to athletic solutions.

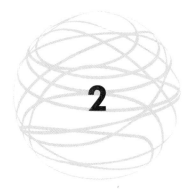

2

Energy as the Problem
and the Antidote

If you run your race, you'll win...
channel your energy.

—Carl Lewis, American track and field athlete;
winner of nine Olympic gold medals

I get up at 4:30 a.m. every day to run my dogs in a fenced-in park. I have to drive there. What with my bleary eyes, we're fortunate that I don't run us off the road. I started this habit because my baseball son got up super early in high school to work out, and in order to wake him, I had to rise earlier than he did. The habit stuck.

Because of my early bird status, it was no big deal for me to meet a young pitcher and his coach at 6 o'clock one summer morning at a facility. The pitcher was struggling to inch up—or I should say "miles-per-hour up"—his velocity. The coach and the pitcher both wanted my input.

After watching the young man throw a few pitches, I stopped him. His velocity was averaging around 84 miles per hour, and I could intuitively perceive the reason. There was a big ball of dark energy around his thighs.

Pitchers have to throw from a strong core. To do this, they must access the power in their hips. But something—some sort of energy—was preventing him from doing this. Intuitively I received a strong sense of the cause of that darkness.

"Your ancestors," I shared. "You are being pulled back by issues related to your ancestry."

He stared at me and then laughed. Apparently, many of his relatives, going back two generations at least, had wanted to play professional baseball. Some were even offered the opportunity, but since pro ball didn't pay well, they'd refused. Their own lost dreams had energetically transformed into a sort of "ball and chain" on my client.

Using a couple of easy techniques, which you'll learn in chapter 4, we cleared the heavy energy. The boy's next pitch registered 8 miles per hour faster.

The truth is that there are lots of different types of energies that can block an athlete. As you learn about these energies and the reasons they occur, start to pay attention to what might explain your athletic performance or what's going on with the athlete in your life.

When Energy Blocks Us

The term "energy blocks" is one that energy medicine practitioners use all the time. Energy blocks are basically problems caused by negative energies, both physical and subtle. I'm going to use that term throughout this book, too, because it's so pictorial and relatable.

Blocks get in the way of our enjoyment of a sport and life itself. This short exercise will help you find a block by feeling it in your body.

EXERCISE 2: FINDING A BLOCK

Think about a time when you were trying to perform your sport—or coach an athlete in their sport—and couldn't pull it off. Return consciously to that experience. You are there again.

Sense the clothes you're wearing, the sounds that surround you, and the smells in the air. Now focus on the task ahead. You're getting *ready, set*—but you can't *go.*

Before you start judging yourself, drop deeper into your body. What do you sense? What is happening? Is there a congested or empty area somewhere inside? Is there an area that feels too tight or too loose? After scanning your body, expand beyond it. Let your sense of self spread way beyond your physical perimeter. Does anything around you draw your attention, such as a pressure, a sensation, or even a being or a person?

Through this assessment, you begin to become aware of an energy that seems to be the problem. That is the block.

We've all experienced a nonstarter, whether while performing or preparing to perform—and probably at all sorts of other times too. While we might have been able to pinpoint the physical cause, there is *always* a subtle reason as well.

That's right: either the energetic data inside or outside you is off or the vibration is wacky or both. Subtle energies organize physical energies. Even if something is wrong physically, at least one of the underlying causes of that physical condition will be a subtle one. That's because the subtle organizes the physical. And this means that to create the most optimum change, you have to focus on the subtle energetics involved in the situation.

This formula doesn't exclude making physical repairs. Imagine you wake up with a horrible headache on one of those important days. Go ahead: take a pain reliever, do a few stretches, breathe deeply, and maybe you'll get through it. Then again, let's say you consistently wake up with a headache every time you need to give a good showing, and none of your physical solutions work.

Which subtle energies might be stuck or unavailable? There are nearly unlimited numbers of answers, but I'm going to help you deep-dive by sharing all the different types of causal issues that could be in play.

A Primer on Energetic Blocks: The Levels of the Self

Blocks can occur within any of the main levels of the self, of which there are four major aspects. Actually, if you think about it, having four parts of yourself is not such a wild idea. Think of how many "selves" you reference on a regular basis:

- ► My body is sore.
- ► My mind is numb.
- ► My soul is on fire.
- ► My spirit is flying high.

These four aspects of you have to be coordinated—or in flow—to give you your best performance. Any or all of them can also be the root of a problem. That means that if you can't find the cause of a block in a single aspect, you'll need to search in others.

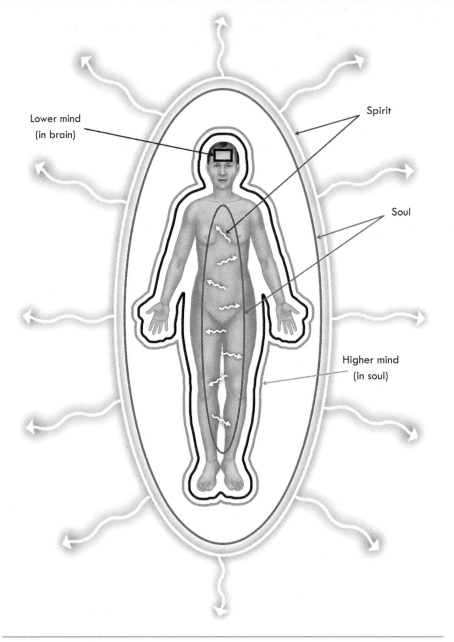

Figure 1: The Four Parts of the Self. We are composed of four main parts of the self. Energy blocks, the causes of our athletic problems, can originate in any of these. The body is the prime vehicle for action. The higher mind holds beliefs and memories and is in the soul. The lower mind is an extension of the soul's mind but is in the brain. The soul is the part of you that travels across time to gain learning. It is supposed to be inside and around the body. Your spirit is your divine spark. It is deep inside and around all other parts of you and is also connected to the greater universe.

Take a look at figure 1, which showcases the four parts of the self in relation to one another.

Your spirit completely surrounds and infuses all other aspects of you. This is your divine spark, and it is entirely pure and wholesome. I like to picture a spirit as the bright light at the end of a sun's ray. That sun is the Source, which some call God and others Allah, the Divine, Kwan Yin, the Goddess, or some other name. I'm going to use the term Higher Power or the Spirit in this book.

Your spirit is always interconnected with the Spirit—and the spirits of all others, alive and dead. It cannot be injured or hurt. Because of this, you'll usually attune to this self for your athletic endeavors.

Your spirit is fully embodied within and around your body and is also connected to all good beings and energies throughout the universe.

Your soul is your spirit's vehicle for moving through time to gain experiences. I visualize it as within and around the body, wrapped inside and nourished by the spirit. Unlike the spirit, your soul can be wounded and make mistakes.

Your soul's job is to experience love while contributing its unique abilities to the world. What does it long for? To leave the world changed in some special way. How you'll accomplish that in a lifetime is called your "soul purpose." In order to fulfill its purpose, the soul undergoes one life after another.

As I said earlier, I believe in reincarnation. When I was a little girl, I remembered having been alive during other times. Funnily, Gabe once asked me if I remembered when he was the big brother and I was the little sister. He remarked, "I had to carry you around all of the time, and you were *really* heavy."

It's important to consider the possibility that you've been incarnate before, as I have found that many athletes' issues are brought in from a different life.

Once a soul finishes with a lifetime, it records everything that happened in the life it has just lived so it can carry all that experience into the next life. Included are memories, feelings, and incomplete teachings. Sometimes our athletic challenges are triggers of a situation that still lingers in our soul.

Let's say that when you're stressed, you can't get your knee to operate correctly. Is that simply a mental concern or a physical malady? You might be retriggering a trauma from a different lifetime. If that's the case, you need to work through the past-life issue in order to work through today's situation.

Your mind is a storage unit of your thoughts and beliefs. The higher mind is actually like a library for your soul. It stores the conclusions you made about circumstances during all lifetimes, and even when you were in between lifetimes. These ideas are transferred into the brain to assist you during a new lifetime. That means you could call your brain your "lower mind."

In this chapter, we'll talk about the nature of thoughts and how they can help you or trip you up. Thoughts are just opinions, but when you're trying to be successful, if you empower the wrong ones, you can easily fall down the rabbit hole. For instance, imagine that during a past life you became convinced that no matter how hard you tried, you'd always lose. Wow! That's going to cause you some problems now in an athletic discipline, isn't it? You have to change the deepest and oldest thoughts that are leading you astray to become successful at your sport—or at just about anything else, for that matter.

Your body is your instrument for moving through this lifetime. If your spirit interacts with it, it will be at its healthiest and most hale. Same if it's affected by the most uplifting parts of your soul or the most supportive and truthful beliefs in your higher and lower mind.

However, your body is vulnerable to negative influences from the soul and the mind, and of course the events of this life, starting with conception.

Think you're merely floating around inside that womb? Nope. You are absorbing everything from your mother's thoughts and feelings to what's happening in the world around her. Not only is your body continually storing externally originated physical energies, but it's a super sponge for subtle energies. Every event that occurs, what you see, feel, touch, experience, and more: all of these are programmed into the body and can affect you positively, neutrally, or negatively.

Think your tendency toward ankle injuries is because you work too much? Maybe. Then again, you might have been standing funny on your ankle when your parents got into a huge argument, and that's the real reason your ankle always turns.

Sometimes an athletic challenge is carried in the body, mind, and soul. Though our spirit doesn't have any issues, it might need to lend its intelligence to our healing process. As an example, I once worked with Ray, a marathon runner who had quit competing because a couple of years earlier his stomach started to knot up when he got near the finale. No matter how hard he tried, he couldn't push through.

I asked what had occurred a couple of years before this started to happen. Apparently, Ray and his husband had adopted a little baby boy. I knew that my client was thrilled about being a father—no problem there—so we probed a little further.

First, I had him rule out issues that could be purely bodily based. Medical tests couldn't find a single problem.

Next, we worked on his childhood. I usually consider this-life events as a part of the this-life body. At age two in this lifetime, Ray's mother had yelled at him and told him that he was worthless, insisting, "Not even God could love you." This statement had landed in his stomach area. As you'll learn, this is the home of the third chakra, which holds our beliefs. The self-perceptions stored there are especially strong. Adopting the child—who was two years old—had triggered my client's issue when he was the same age. This discovery showed that his lower mind (or brain) was also involved.

Even though Ray worked through this event, he still couldn't reach the finish line. So we had to probe his soul.

During a regression, Ray remembered being a woman who had died in childbirth. When separating from this body at death, he was so dismayed and upset that he decided to never trust God (the word he used for Higher Power) again. After all, what kind of God would take a mother from her child?

Underneath this reaction was a higher-mind belief that he didn't deserve to be loved and protected by God. At this point we called on Ray's spirit, which showed him that God had never abandoned him. Ray's soul decided it was willing to let God in again—and just like that, the soul, lower mind, higher mind, and childhood issue shifted. So did his third chakra and his body. After retraining for a few months, he was back to his marathons, all the way to the finish line.

As you're probably perceiving, there could be a lot of reasons why you don't reach your performance aims, but most of them will come down to a single idea: trauma.

EXERCISE 3: ARE YOU DEALING WITH TRAUMA?

Reflect on the following questions, either in regard to yourself or an athlete you care about, and see what strikes you.

In regard to sports, do you believe…

- ▸ You are not living up to your potential?
- ▸ You are stuck on a hamster wheel?

- You should "make it"—whatever that means to you—but can tell something is in the way?
- You are more scared of succeeding than failing?
- You are scared because you keep failing when you should be succeeding?
- Something external is blocking you from moving forward?
- You are powerless to change?
- Something inside of you is preventing forward movement?

If so, you are probably dealing with the residuals of trauma. Trauma can cause all of these effects:

- Block optimum performance.
- Create confusion about what preparation to do.
- Keep you from getting out of bed to do what you should.
- Lead to your being injury prone.
- Stop you from appropriately caring for an injury.
- Slow injury recovery.
- Cause self-sabotage.
- Turn a mere slip into a serious downward spiral.
- Force mental and emotional mayhem.
- Convince you that you don't have trauma.

It's All About Trauma

Trauma is stress that fails to clear.

Everything about life is stressful. There are negative, positive, and neutral stressors, but in the end, the only thing that matters is your reaction to a stressor, not what anyone else thinks of it.

A *stressor* is an event that causes imbalance. Pretty much anything that makes you regroup in order to reach a new state of equilibrium or balance, consciously or unconsciously, is a stressor. As is implied, a stressor can involve any of the four parts of the self, if not all of them. I'll give you a simple example of a bodily stress that includes emotional challenges.

I worked with a young college student who loved to work out. In fact, his workouts were key to his keeping a strong B average. Joe didn't play on a team. He worked out alone. So, was he an athlete? He saw himself as such and constantly wanted to improve. That meant that his "game day" was the day he lifted a heavier weight or accomplished a particular movement he'd been aiming for.

Over the last year, Joe's training had gone by the wayside because his girlfriend was becoming increasingly needy. Every time he had to spend a night studying, she broke down emotionally. If he Snapchatted with a woman friend, she accused him of cheating. She would show up at his apartment at night to search the place for another woman. When he wanted to spend time with his family, she screamed that she was being cut out.

Obviously, she needed therapeutic help. Joe also needed assistance, though, because the pressure was keeping him from feeling good enough about himself to keep up his exercise routine—or to deal with the real question: Did he want to stay in the relationship or not?

I explained to Joe that he was in a traumatizing relationship, and that continual emotional and verbal pressure has a physical effect, for sure, but also a subtle one. Essentially, when his girlfriend was shaming him, she was simultaneously stealing his life energy. *Life energy* is our electrical and chemical energy. It is generated by our first chakra, which you'll learn more about in the next chapter. Located in the base of the spine, this chakra generates the energy needed for our physicality.

Besides being drained of life energy, Joe was also taking on his girlfriend's issues and feelings. As you'll also learn, we can bring the energies of other people into ourselves, which can cause serious problems in our bodily self.

After understanding what was occurring on the subtle energetic level, Joe was ready to change this pattern.

It wasn't an easy breakup. He needed several weeks to build up his courage to do it, and then to keep resisting her manipulation in the aftermath. During that time, however, he was able to begin following a healthy nutritional program. Gradually, he returned to the gym. It took him six months to completely reengage with his program, but that's okay.

Joe's athleticism had been broken by current-day trauma. Look at how it impacted everything about his physical sportiness. He had to patiently rebuild his sense of self along with his physical capabilities, but he did it.

At one level, Joe's trauma was relatively easy to deal with. I say that because it was more bodily than mind or soul based, although he was seriously impacted by what I'd call lower mind beliefs such as "You have to take what people dish out." As well, his stressors, and therefore trauma, were relatively recent. I've found that the older the traumatic events are, the harder it is to work through them.

In addition, Joe was "only" dealing with a specific type of trauma—psychological. That can be a horrific challenge, but there are many other origins of stress that can result in trauma, as I'll explain.

A Model for Trauma: The Root of All Athletic Difficulties

As I've explained, trauma starts with stressors, and stress affects us both physically and subtly. To help you really understand what might be causing a negative impact on your athleticism, I'm going to walk you through the three main stages of trauma: stress in the physical body, stress in the subtle body, and then the locking-in of these stressors in both the physical and subtle bodies.

Stress in the Physical Body

On the physical level, a stressor sets off a bodily reaction. This might clear; then again, it can anchor for the long term. What's actually happening inside of us? I'll lay it out.

The bone marrow produces osteocalcin. This busy little hormone says *red alert!* as it travels through the body.

The nervous system goes into overdrive—and boy, does it. I'm going to highlight just a few of the many circumstances that occur as a result.

First off, the nervous system issues a stream of stress hormones. Some of the main ones include adrenaline and cortisol, which are made by the adrenals. These and other little reactionaries raise your heart rate and blood pressure, quicken your breathing, tighten your muscles, close off your digestive system, make you sweat, and so much more.

In particular, the polyvagal nervous system kicks in. This is a very important part of your entire nervous system. Its main constituent is the vagus nerve, which is one of the many cranial nerves. Passing downward through the body from the neck area, this nerve connects pretty much all your organs (and chakras, by the way) to each other. This nerve is one of the most critical to your health and athletic ability.

The vagus nerve is socially programmed. That means it holds all your conscious and unconscious ideas about how to be safe and fit in. If you fall apart when someone is negative about your performance, it's probably because your vagus nerve says you should. If you had a coach who yelled all the time—or you had a parent who always yelled at games—your vagus nerve might make you yell at yourself if you screw up.

The polyvagal system runs your autonomic nervous system, which manages your internal system and processes. There are three main parts within it. Each is highly complicit in stress and locked-in trauma.

- *Sympathetic nervous system:* This autonomic branch makes the excitable hormones that get you going—and run the fright, flight, fight, and fawn stress reactions.

- *Parasympathetic nervous system:* This branching system relaxes you and sort of puts you on vacation in Mexico at the beach.

- *Enteric nervous system:* This is also called the "second" and "gut" brain and is a collection of neurotransmitters in the abdominal area that pretty much manages all of your feelings, in addition to your stress reactions, digestive processes, and immune system. In fact, 80 percent of your immune health is based on the healthiness or lack thereof in this region. That vagus nerve? About 90 percent of its communications run from your gut to your head brain, not the other way around. With more neurotransmitters than are found in the brain, this region determines much of your athletic expertise, activity habits, emotional issues, mental patterns, and ability to repair from injury, so yup—we'll be working with this part of your body a lot!

Your thalamus throws you into shock. This is a small organ in the brain. Along with other parts of you, it sends the just-engaged, stressed self into a state of shock. This is so you can respond to events without letting pesky feelings or problems get in the way.

Your ancestors start voting. What? Physically, your genetic material is surrounded by a chemical soup called the epigenome. In this soup are at least fourteen generations of your ancestors' memories, ready to be triggered and inform you of how to act, feel, and think. Imprinted are the events that happened to your ancestors and—equally important—their reactions to those events. When a situation in your own life is similar to one in an ancestor's life, the chemicals in the epigenome can end up taking over.

That might be great if an ancestral imprint jumps in helpfully. Let's say your great-grandpa was terrific under pressure. You'll probably have a super beneficial reaction when under stress too. But let's say that he used to quit under pressure. Guess what you might do?

Aftermath. Once the crisis is over, your body is supposed to relax. You stop pumping out excitatory hormones. You exit shock and deal with your feelings. You problem-solve and readjust—unless you don't leave that stress behind and it doesn't leave you.

Stress in the Subtle Body

How does your subtle self react to a stressor? Well, this is interesting stuff.

There are actually five main topics to understand regarding the subtle system and stress: *forces*, *negative subtle charges*, *energetic constructs*, *ancestral and soul issues*, and the *shock bubble*.

I know that's a mouthful. Stay with me and I'll share not only what all of this means, but why it's so important to understand in regard to sports.

1: Forces Are What Cause the Stress

A force is a field or wave of energy that causes an impact. While you can perceive the effects of a force, you can't see forces with your physical eyes. But if you pay attention, you'll realize that every interaction in life is a product of a force or forces. If someone kisses you, the kiss is planted through a force. If a ball hits you on the head, that's a force that causes a response.

There are six basic types of forces, and each of these can create stress or imbalance.

Physical forces: These impact you through a physical interaction that causes a response. Examples include getting hit, falling, being slammed around, or getting sick. Physical forces underlie many athletic injuries, from torn muscles to traumatic brain injuries, but they aren't all bad. They can also support an athlete. I was watching an American football game where a young man caught a pass and then fumbled it right on the three-yard line. Just then, an opposing teammate stumbled into him and he recaught the fumble and scored a touchdown. That particular physical force actually helped the team score!

Environmental forces: These forces are initiated by the environment. Think of the harm created by climactic changes such as tornadoes, hurricanes, or the like. There are conditions that generate negative reactions in certain athletes, depending on their history. I worked with a bobsledder whose parents had died during a winter storm. After that happened, every time snow fell, his performance fell apart. That pattern obviously didn't serve him, so we worked to shift it by using techniques you'll learn in this book.

Emotional forces: There are various types of psychological forces. One of them is emotional. An emotion is a feeling plus a belief. We create emotions all the time, for they enable us to get through an event, respond accurately, and figure out what we need. If a bee comes after us, our thought is *This bee can hurt me.* The feeling is probably fear. The combination of that belief and that feeling is enough to get us to move—fast.

An emotional force, however, comprises a belief and a feeling that come at us with intensity. If someone is watching our performance and thinking it's awful and is angry with us for making them look bad, we'll pick up on that force, and it can impact us.

An emotional force might or might not include a verbal force. Verbal forces often contain a belief, feeling, or both, and they can be beneficial or injurious. If someone is yelling from the bleachers *You can do it!* and they mean it, that might boost our abilities. But if someone is screaming *You're blowing it,* that verbal force can injure our self-perception enough to cause us to lose focus.

Because we're talking subtle energies, know that you can be wounded by a psychological force that isn't shared aloud. We've all felt a coach or parent thinking negatively about us, and it hurts, doesn't it?

I have a client whose pitching was fantastic on all the teams he played on except his college team. Guess what? He knew the pitching coach didn't like him, and he could feel it as soon as he stepped on the mound.

Digital forces: These days, digital media can deliver either uplifting or damaging forces. When social media reactions are positive, we feel good. But that dig about our performance on social media, the nasty email, ghosting on a dating site—all of these and more can cause harm. For athletes, sometimes all it takes is a cutting comment from someone who's following your training practices to undercut your performance, at least in the short term.

Spiritual forces: These forces are a cornucopia of invisible sources of energy that can create negative influences. This list includes ghosts, deceased ancestors, and negative entities and energies. These often link with us through energetic constructs that are covered in point 3 of this section. Spiritual forces can drain us or fill us with others' negative energies.

Missing forces: This is a really important force. Ironically, although it doesn't exist, I think it's the cause of many athletic issues. A missing force is one that should have been given to us but wasn't. I'll give you an example.

When we're young, we thrive best in our athletic endeavors with the support and care of at least one parental figure. One year my youngest was on a truly Bad News Bears team. They lost absolutely every game—and I'm talking by at least twenty runs—until after the Fourth of July. I'll never figure out what was so magical about America's Independence Day, but that was when they finally started to win.

One young boy—I'll call him Jasper—was always brought to games by his mom and grandpa. I never saw his father. Jasper hadn't had a hit until July 4, and then he suddenly became the top scorer. He remained a steady Eddie until early August, when his father finally came to a game. When Jasper was up, he stood at the plate, swung, and missed. Not only once but twice and then three times. He struck out. His father shook his head and left, and Jasper cried in the dugout.

The lack of parental support qualified as a missing force for Jasper, so much so that when his father came to a game, he couldn't even hit the ball.

To really understand how a force impacts us, there are several correlating factors. These are the existence of entrance and exit points, stuck points, and pathways.

Entrance points: Wherever the force hits or first interacts with us is its entrance point. Did you get bonked on the head with a volleyball? The site of that injury is the entrance point. Did the ball simply brush your energetic field without touching your body? Even if the point of contact is external (outside your physical body), it qualifies as an entrance point. That area is prime for further problems, from causing physical weakness to becoming a site for built-up repressed feelings.

Exit points: If the force passes all the way through (or across) the body and then leaves you, that area is the exit point. Exit points often qualify as injury sites but can be very hard to identify because the exit point isn't always found directly across from the entrance site. If a force enters at an angle, the exit point will be found in relationship to that angle.

Many exit points are found directly across from entrance points, however. For instance, I once worked with a professional ballerina who had broken her right arm. It was healing well, but she couldn't figure out why her left arm also hurt all the time.

It turned out that the physical force that broke her right arm went straight through the body and exited the left arm, so it was getting sore as well. I worked with a former football player, though, who had once had a concussion at the top right area of his head. It was an obvious entrance point, as he'd been hit in the head there. He didn't know why his left foot hurt all the time too. That was actually the exit point, as the ball had entered at an angle.

Stuck points: Sometimes a force doesn't leave the body. Rather, it gets stuck there. That jammed place often experiences problems, from emotional residue to tumors or internal pains.

Pathways: As has been implied, this is the trajectory between any entrance or exit/stuck point. The pathway can often cause problems, primarily because of the next point I'm going to make.

When an athlete has been injured by a force, we often determine the entrance site, which can be anything from the energy field to a chakra to a part of the body. We also look for the pathway and any stuck or exit points. But there is another factor that is equally vital, if not more so, in its impact.

2: Negative Subtle Charges

Negative subtle charges create more stress. Dealing with a force is tough enough, but there is another problem associated with forces that's even more serious. Forces can often transfer negative subtle charges into our system.

Negative subtle charges are just that: subtle energies that are "charged" with information that is detrimental to us. They can also be vibrating at frequencies that are bad for us. Whatever doesn't match our "real self" can create damage.

From a scientific point of view, atoms can carry an electrical or magnetic charge. So can subtle energies. But when I apply the word *negative*, I mean something different from the polarity of a charge. I'm talking about a subtle energy that holds an imprint, or someone else's energy, that is harmful. Once these subtle charges enter us, they can litter the pathway or get anchored in an entrance, exit, or stuck point.

We can't process energies that aren't our own. So, for example, if a force transfers into us someone else's anger, bitterness, or even the energy of an illness, that energy can remain in our body and create reactivity that includes physical and psychological reactions.

Think about it. Maybe someone has flung a shaming comment to you, loudly, something like "I can't believe you were so stupid that you did that!" That screaming constitutes a psychological force, both emotional and verbal. If you think about a comment like that and still feel a reaction, such as the feeling of shame, those subtle charges might still be stuck in your system. And there they sit, potentially making you think you are too stupid to change your mechanics, meet your objectives, or hold your own—or something equally damaging.

Some subtle charges can be positive. I have worked with one professional weightlifting athlete who always talks with his dad right before he competes. "I can feel his good energy over the phone," shared the athlete. Another personal coach who consults with me about his athletes says he texts each of them before an important event because he knows his "vote" can make all the difference.

3: Energetic Constructs

Energetic constructs get hooked into the stress. Stress can create connections—or stir up already existing ones—that are negative and energetic in nature. I'm talking about something called *energetic constructs.*

Also called *contracts*, these are subtle energy bindings that restrict activity, physical and emotional health, spiritual powers, and even destiny. All parts of the body, mind, and soul, as well as the subtle energy anatomy, are susceptible to these bindings, which can remain in place during a part or the entirety of a lifetime or from lifetime to lifetime. They can exist between any two people or beings or among a group. And by beings, I mean natural beings, like animals, or entities, which are souls that are either living or dead. They can also link us to dark forces, which are really bad and conscious beings that cause great harm, often supporting racism, sexism, ageism, genocide, and other major destructive conflicts.

There are two basic types of subtle constructs. There are *attachments,* which serve as unhealthy linkages, and *holds,* which basically reduce the level of success that a victim of a hold can achieve.

A lot of athletic problems originate in these types of issues. I'm just going to cover a few of them and provide a couple of examples. You'll start learning how to deal with them in chapter 4.

Energetic Attachments: There are three main types of these that can really create damage in the athlete: *cords, curses*, and *energy markers*. An attachment can get carried in on a force or get stirred by one.

- ▸ Cords are like garden hoses through which energy flows, and they may appear that way intuitively. Often we find ourselves taking on others' issues, emotions, or pain through a cord in exchange for giving them our healthy energies. I had a client who struggled during tournaments that his father attended. He had a difficult relationship with his father. He could literally feel his father's emotions enter his chest and his own life energy drain out, exiting through the first chakra. Before we worked on the issue, he had to go so far as to ask his father not to attend his important games.

- ► Curses are tube-shaped bundles of cords that bunch together and cause a repetitive event or the lack of one. For instance, you can inherit a curse passed down from one or both sides of your family or be cursed—deliberately or not—by a person or a group. I worked with a woman who had just quit participating in tournaments for older-age downhill skiers because every time she won, horrors befell her. Once, her son got in an accident; another time, she became violently ill. We tracked it to a curse put on her by a jealous sister. We cleared it, and she was able to happily compete again.

- ► Energy markers look like clumps of swirling charges moving counterclockwise and forming a symbol, usually an X. This symbol will "instruct" others in how to treat the marker. For instance, an energy marker was causing one of my athlete clients to go unnoticed by scouts, even though he was the best player on the team. We cleared the energy marker, and he began to get accolades.

Energetic Holds: These energetic bindings restrict the full functioning of their victims. For instance, many parents put holds on their children, sometimes to keep them safe, but sometimes to ensure that the child takes care of them (the parent). Types of holds include the following:

- ► Deflection shields. These psychically invisible sheaths deflect a particular form of goodness. For an athlete, these can be very challenging. What if you are wearing an armor you can't see that rejects attention or being picked for the team or the fulfillment of some other need?

▶ Miasms. This is an energetic field that programs a group of souls or family members; miasms often create psychological, physical, and spiritual disease patterns within family systems. You might carry a failure miasm from one or both sides of your family. That can cause you to literally "strike out" when you don't want to.

4: Ancestral and Soul Issues

Ancestral and soul issues might kick in. We've already discussed the presence of an epigenome in our physical body that holds our ancestral memories. And several times I've discussed the soul, which carries experiences from one lifetime to another. Well, I'm creating a placeholder here for the athlete who can't figure out where their issues come from. A stressor can easily trigger an ancestor's issues, as well as an experience held within your soul. Sometimes both occur.

I worked with a professional golfer who froze during every tournament. He'd yet to place, which meant his income was pretty darn low; in fact, he made his living giving golf lessons. Even that profession would have been boosted by a placement.

What did we figure out? Well, we know there aren't a lot of golfers who lived hundreds of years ago, but we did uncover one, using the techniques provided in this book, who was the oldest son of a farmer and inherited the farm when his father died. The rest of his family detested him for his good luck and actually spun a curse on him.

A curse is a statement that comes true. Every time that farmer was on the verge of a healthy crop, a disaster would occur. He could eke out a living, but only just. That farmer? He was both an ancestor of my client's as well as his own soul! Yes, he'd been his own ancestor, which gave the curse a double whammy. The possibility of winning stirred the curse and the gut reaction of guilt. We cleared this—and he placed!

5: Shock Bubble

The shocked self remains stuck. We talked about the fact that under stress, our system goes into shock. Well, that is true. Picture this self as stuck in a bubble. Well, guess what happens if we never get out of that shock bubble? That is the basis for trauma.

The Trauma Model

If you are consistently challenged in one or several ways, you basically remain stuck in a shock bubble. That inner self turns into a trapped self, an injured and wounded self that, unless freed, continually re-experiences the event that caused the original stress. That self will most likely hold two very different opinions about being in this state.

The first is *At least I'm safe inside this bubble.* Thinking that, the shocked self might not present itself for healing. That makes it hard to discover the origin of a challenge with exactness. Then again, this self might think *I want out of here!* To escape, that self hijacks the entire physical and psychological self when situations feel similar to those that caused the original stressor.

Of course, life is ever changing because that bubbled self is still going through the original stressor, keeping the rest of you in the same state. Following are a few indicators of this.

- Your sympathetic nervous system, and other systems, remain in overdrive. If you're always in fright/flight/freeze/fight/fawn mode, you'll be simultaneously wired and continually exhausted. The latter can make it hard to devote yourself to a good workout or another preparation program or remain fixed on your goals. You could become emotionally and mentally oversensitive. You could also find yourself unable to focus and become vulnerable to injury.

- Forces and reactions repeat. If you were originally felled by a particular force or set of forces, you'll keep attracting the same types of forces. It's the same with any lodged negative subtle charges. This complication makes it difficult to pinpoint the original stress so you can clear it and recover.

You never know what you might attract. I'll give you an example.

Years ago, during the year of the Bad News Bears team I mentioned earlier in this chapter, one of the boys (I'll call him Jimmy) had a mother who was scared he would get a concussion. She was so frightened of this that she sat in a tent at the edge of the field during every game, with the tent's opening facing away from the game, as she didn't want to see Jimmy get that I-know-it's-going-to-happen concussion. During one of our last games, the field was configured oddly so there was no place near a street where she could plant her tent. So she had to sit near the rest of the moms in the bleachers. Still, she resided in her tent, which, as expected, faced away from the game.

Jimmy came to bat. The pitcher pitched. Jimmy swung and made contact. *Whap!* The ball flew up and over the fence, curving around to enter Jimmy's mother's tent, only to whonk her on the head.

She was okay, but we found out later that she'd actually had a concussion when she was young. Little wonder she was scared for her son, but at the same time she had attracted a harmful physical force to herself.

- ▸ Eventually you could develop immune challenges, including problems with selecting and digesting healthy foods and difficulties in recovery from injury. If these challenges are advanced, the body will overproduce mast cells: immune cells that, when populated in the body, cause inflammation and stiffness.

- ▸ You'll continue to trigger epigenetic, ancestral responses. That can make it hard for you to know whether you're triggering your own issues or those of your ancestors.

- ▸ Energetic constructs will attract situations and people similar to those that created them. Had an overbearing parent to whom you were or are corded? If the pattern was to take on their problems, you'll do that for an overbearing coach.

With all the issues that could be affecting you and your athleticism, it could feel hard to decide if you are impacted by a traumatic block or something else. The following exercise presents questions that will help you initiate that discussion.

EXERCISE 4: SENSING A TRAUMATIC BLOCK

How do you know if your athletic career or that of an athlete you are working with is affected by a locked-in trauma? I'll repeat the questions I presented earlier, with a number of additional ones. If any or many of these stir a response, you might be dealing with trauma, and you'll want to deal with it.

In regard to sports, do you believe…

- ▸ you aren't living up to your potential?

- ▸ you are stuck on a hamster wheel?

- ▸ you should "make it"—whatever that means to you—but can tell something is in the way?

- ▸ you are more scared of succeeding than failing?

- ▸ you are scared because you keep failing when you should be succeeding?
- ▸ something external is blocking you from moving forward?
- ▸ you are powerless to change?
- ▸ something inside of you is preventing forward movement?
- ▸ that the cause of your challenge is historical?
- ▸ that the reason you can't achieve what you desire lies in your family history?
- ▸ that you've lived before, and you're being impacted by one of those experiences?
- ▸ that there is an invisible energy pulling you backward?
- ▸ that you are acting out someone else's problems?
- ▸ that you are oversensitive to what is occurring around you?

Most athletic challenges are a product of stress that gets locked into the physical and subtle selves, therefore turning into trauma. Trauma is complicated and can result in physical, psychological, and even spiritual challenges, any of which can create difficulties for the athlete. Traumatic events can be rooted in our childhood or adulthood as well as our own past lives and the lives of our ancestors. Because trauma involves the delivery of forces, and quite possibly the transference of negative subtle charges, we often become afflicted by energies that aren't our own. Ultimately, improving our athletic and coaching abilities will be linked to freeing any wounded selves from trauma and clearing forces and negative subtle charges.

All is not lost, of course—this book is here to help you resolve all these conditions! But before you can work on the issues creating your athletic challenges, it's essential to know how the subtle anatomy works, which is the topic of our next chapter.

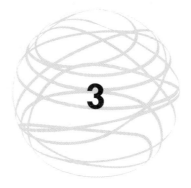

3

Subtle Structures
for Changing Energy

*You have to be able to focus, to control your
energy. You need to make it your ally...*

—Elvis Stojko, Canadian figure skater, two-time
Olympic silver medalist, in *Sports Psychology*

Jonas was an older gentleman who loved karate. In fact, he made a living teaching it—until his chest started to constrict every time he worked up a sweat.

Cleared of physical heart issues, he came to me. "It's got to be energetic," he insisted.

Often, individuals who practice disciplines like yoga and the martial arts are aware of subtle energies, as well as of the subtle anatomy. We soon figured out that Jonas's chest tension had started on the exact month and date when he had lost his own father from a heart attack decades previously.

It took a few sessions to help Jonas deep-dive into the emotional pain left over from his rather empty relationship with his father. What did we focus on? Two things: the shock bubble self and feelings in his fourth chakra, also called the heart chakra. After several sessions, Jonas was able to clear the physical tension when it arose, using breathing techniques such as the four-six breathing exercise featured in chapter 1. He then returned joyfully to his karate endeavors.

How can you facilitate this type of ease using subtle energy tools? Start by learning about the three systems of subtle energy anatomy. Then you enhance that foundation by learning a model that explains how frequencies factor in.

Your Core Subtle Energy Systems

In chapter 1 you learned that there are organs (or centers), channels, and fields in your subtle anatomy, just as there are in your physical body. You also learned that you use your intuition to relate to this subtle anatomy. But you're going to actually meet these subtle systems, starting right now.

The Chakras: Your Major Subtle Centers

Knowledge of the chakras has existed throughout the world for thousands of years. There are differing systems or models, but the shared agreement among the many cultures that use them is that every chakra manages a specific set of physical, psychological, and spiritual functions. For you, this means that if you can track an issue you're having with your athletic performance to a chakra, you can shift the subtle and physical energies that are creating the problem and thereby alleviate it.

The majority of chakras are anchored in a specific set of vertebrae, and all of them relate to an endocrine gland. A chakra also governs the tissues that are connected to it. For instance, the first chakra, located in the hips, operates through the coccygeal vertebrae as well as the main hormone gland associated with that area, the adrenals. Besides this, however, the first chakra engineers the health of the genitals, anus, large intestine, and the other parts of the body found in its geographic territory.

That's the physical aspect of the first chakra. Psychologically, each chakra is activated during a specific age range. That is, it locks in issues that develop during those months or years. That first chakra? It is prime from when you're in the womb until you reach six months of age. During that time period, it's busily absorbing issues about your safety and security and figuring out the main principles of your identity. The subconscious conclusions stored within that chakra will continue to impact all your related issues and decisions, from making money to your physical well-being. (You'll find the ages of activation for each chakra listed in chapter 4.)

Spiritually, each chakra operates on a specific band of frequencies; these can be described as *colors* and *sounds*. This means that a chakra attracts related frequencies from the external world for internal processing, and it also dispenses like-minded messages. This function allows it to be described as an intuitive center. That first chakra? It is physically empathic, letting you sense what is occurring in the external environment and specifically within others' bodies—these are its specialties. We'll more thoroughly examine the intuitive specialties of each chakra further along, also in chapter 4.

While the majority of Westerners use a seven-chakra system, I employ a twelve-chakra system. I developed it decades ago, and it's become a gold standard worldwide. It's interesting to note that the man said to be the creator of the Western seven-chakra system you may have heard of never actually said that there are only seven chakras. In fact, he presented six chakras and an extra energy body! He also indicated that there are dozens of chakra systems in India alone, the geographic source of his model, and it's vital to figure out which works for you.

I use a twelve-chakra system because when I was a child, I could see those twelve orbs of light around my family members. Once I learned that I was perceiving chakras (the word didn't exist in the white Wonder Bread Norwegian Lutheran family I grew up in), I conducted personal and cross-cultural research to showcase all twelve chakras. I love working with the "extra" five chakras because these afford a greater range of interactions and much more powerful and precise energy work.

The twelve chakras—and what each one manages—are depicted on figure 2.

The Structure of the Chakras

If you become a chakra expert—and I hope you do, at least in relation to your own chakras—you'll need to understand the structure of chakras. In fact, using your intuition, which you'll be prompted to start doing in chapter 4, will be easier if you first comprehend the structure.

Looking at it simplistically, there are two mechanical properties of chakras to be aware of.

Inner and Outer Wheels: That's right—chakras are shaped like wheels. Each has an internal wheel and an external wheel. Picture a donut. The outside wheel is the cake part, the ring around the hole. The internal wheel is the hole.

The external wheel holds all our worldly programs. These can consist of programs or ideas related to your soul and ancestral issues, family of origin ideas and experiences, and all the beliefs you've created in your life throughout adulthood (if you are there yet!). Basically, if something is going wrong, the belief system related to that is carried on the outside wheels.

Chakra 1
(1) Red
(2) Hips
(3) Coccygeal vertebrae, adrenals
(4) Hips area, genitals, large
intestine, anus, rectum
(5) Safety and security
(6) In utero to 6 months
(7) Physical empathy
and manifesting

Chakra 2
(1) Orange
(2) Abdomen
(3) Sacral vertebrae
and ovaries or testes
(4) Sacrum area, small intestine,
sexual organs and their functions
(5) Emotions and creativity
(6) 6 months to 2½ years
(7) Feeling empathy
and creativity

Chakra 3
(1) Yellow
(2) Solar plexus
(3) Thorasic vertebrae
and pancreas
(4) Most digestive organs
(5) Power and self-esteem
(6) 2½ to 4½ years
(7) Cognitive empathy and
administrative functions

Chakra 5
(1) Blue
(2) Throat
(3) Cervical vertebrae and thyroid
(4) All glands and body parts
associated with throat, neck, jaws, teeth
(5) Expression and communication
(6) 6½ to 8½ years
(7) Clairaudience, or
"clear hearing"

Chakra 6
(1) Violet
(2) Brow
(3) Higher vertebrae, pituitary gland
(4) All body parts related to eyes,
seeing, overseeing, or hormones
and parts of brain
(5) Self-image and goal setting
(6) 8½ to 14 years
(7) Clairvoyance, or
"clear seeing"

Chakra 7
(1) White
(2) Top of head/
inside center of head
(3) Cranial area, pineal gland
(4) Brain learning centers,
cranium and cranium bones
(5) Spirituality and life purpose
(6) 14 to 21 years
(7) Prophecy, or clear
consciousness

Chakra 9
(1) Gold
(2) A foot over the head
(3) Diaphragm
(4) Breathing functions; holds codes
to assist all parts of the body
(5) Harmony with others
(6) 28 to 35 years
(7) Ability to harmonize

Chakra 10
(1) Brown
(2) A foot under the feet
(3) Bone marrow
(4) All bone functions,
genes, and epigenetics
(5) Place in the world,
relationship with Nature
(6) Pre-conception, conception;
also 35 to 42 years
(7) Natural empathy

Chakra 11
(1) Pink
(2) In the energy field, also
around the hands and feet
(3) Connective tissue
(4) Muscles, connective tissue, collagen
(5) Connectivity with others
(6) 42 to 49 years
(7) Commanding of supernatural
and natural forces

Chakra 4

(1) Green

(2) Chest

(3) Cardiac plexus and heart

(4) All organs in chest, ribs

(5) Love and relationship

(6) 4½ to 6½ years

(7) Relational empathy
and healing powers

Chakra 8

(1) Black/Silver

(2) An inch above the head

(3) Thymus

(4) Immune system

(5) Sense of self as mystical

(6) 21 to 28 years

(7) All mystical and
shamanic abilities

Chakra 12

(1) Clear or opaque

(2) Outer rim of auric
field; can also be accessed
in center of fourth chakra

(6) Chakra 12, which develops between
49 and 56 years of age, is unique to
each person and holds your own special
intuitive gifts; after age 56, the chakras
begin to recycle in seven-year
blocks, and you start over
again with the first
chakra.

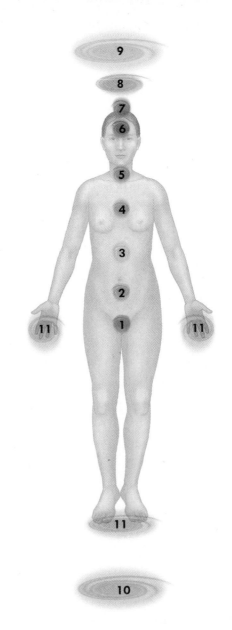

Figure 2: The Twelve-Chakra System. Each chakra can be described with specific attributes. In this illustration you will find the following factors: (1) chakra color, (2) location, (3) spinal area and/or endocrine gland, (4) primary physical functions, (5) primary psychological ideas, (6) age of development, and (7) intuitive gifts. The twelfth chakra is not pictured here. (See the special insert for a colorized version.)

The internal wheel contains your spirit energy, as well as the energy from your Higher Power or Higher Spirit. I always ask people to center themselves in this inner wheel when doing their energetic work.

Front and Back Sides: The front of a chakra is the part that faces forward in relation to your spine. The back side faces back, behind you. The front side looks into your future and receives impressions from it. The back side receives information from your past and your unconscious, as well as spiritual energies. When dealing with downward spirals, you'll learn how important it is to be centered in the spine, not shifted either forward or backward. We'll also apply other concepts to this structure.

Energetic Blocks and the Chakras

As we discussed in the previous chapter, an energetic block affecting your athletics might originate in the body, mind, or soul. It could relate to this life or another one, or it could be a multigenerational issue, and it will most likely involve a trauma of some sort. There are so many possibilities for what might cause a problem that it's extremely helpful to have a single place to start working in—like a chakra.

A lot of times I find that a struggling athlete is blocked in their first chakra, one of the most crucial for athletes. Of course, right? That's the chakra that manages our overall physical health and even our sense of worthiness. What factors could be more prime for an athlete than those?

I once worked with a hockey player who kept throwing out his hip at the worst of times. When he was ready to pop the puck into the net, Jamal's hips would freeze. His doctor had ruled out a physical condition, so it was up to me to probe the energetics.

As you can see in figure 2, the hips relate to the first chakra. The first chakra develops from the time in the womb to six months of age. With that in mind, Jamal combed his memories for first chakra issues—and remembered his mother telling him that he had been born with a twisted leg and a broken hip. That type of physical trauma, involving a physical force, could certainly underlie his hip symptoms. There were also indications of stuck subtle charges, however.

Jamal had a talk with his mother to ask if there were any difficult emotional issues involved in his birth. Her answer brought her to tears. She and his father had discussed getting divorced, and then she became pregnant. Jamal's father agreed to stay only until the child was born, and in fact, my client's parents had divorced by the time he was two years old.

It made sense to me that Jamal's mother's distress, along with his father's reluctance and resentment, formulated negative subtle charges that locked into his hips. At an unconscious level, that baby felt responsible for both parents' feelings and their doomed marriage. Because of that burden, Jamal simply didn't feel that he deserved success.

It took a while, as we were working with preverbal issues, but Jamal reconciled them and cleared the stuck force and negative charges. His hip stopped locking up.

The Subtle Energy Channels

Think of chakras as islands, each pulsing with specific types of power that can enable athletic prowess. Flowing through and around these isles are riverways of light and sound: the energy channels.

There are two basic types of subtle energy channels. The *nadis* are comparable to your nerves. They are the main energy channels depicted in Hindu systems and allow an activation and spread of electrical energy. Every part of you pulses with electricity, and if you have enough of it flowing through your nadis, or nerves, you'll be balanced on all levels. The nadis also carry life energy, which supports the chakras.

I often assist with clearing and activating the nadis if an athlete is lacking in physical energy or is feeling off mentally or emotionally. You'll learn an exercise in chapter 9, Stimulating Your Vagus Nerve, to help you do the same. It works on the nadis as well as the vagus nerve because the nadis are essentially the nervous system, and the vagus nerve is the head of that organ system. Also, in chapter 4, exercise 15, you'll be given the opportunity to adjust the nadis along with other subtle body components.

The other major energy channels are the meridians. *Meridian* is the term used in traditional Chinese medicine and other Eastern modalities to reference pathways of energy that feed the entire body. The major meridians, which number twelve, flow through your connective tissue and have been scientifically found to carry electrical charges. Each meridian is headed by an organ, such as the liver or the spleen, and regulates specific physical, psychological, and spiritual functions. They can be accessed through acupoints, which are invisible entry sites on the skin. Meridian-based therapies such as acupuncture have been shown to be quite calming, balancing, and clearing.

Auric Field	Color
First	Red
Tenth	Brown
Second	Orange
Third	Yellow
Fourth	Green
Fifth	Blue
Sixth	Violet
Seventh	White
Eighth	Black
Ninth	Gold
Eleventh	Pink
Twelfth	Translucent

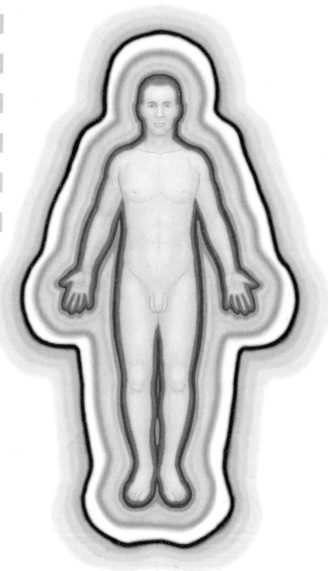

Figure 3: The Twelve Auric Layers. The auric field is composed of twelve individual fields or layers, each of which extends from a chakra. Each field is the same color as—and communicates with—its associated chakra. The fields are atop each other in the same numerical order as the chakras except for the tenth field, which lies between the first and second fields. The first field is the closest to the body. (See the special insert for a colorized version.)

The Auric Layers/Fields

Every chakra oscillates with light and sound waves, which creates a field of light and sound extending outside the body. Every single chakra turns into its own field, and together they form the overall auric field. These various layers operate like external guards for their related chakras. They determine which energies will be allowed in, for example, and they send subtle messages into the world. Their decisions, however, are determined by the chakras, which store all your programs, or internal beliefs.

As we've shared, the first chakra holds programs related to safety and security. These programs operate like the software running the hardware of your body. They also regulate the protective tasks of the first auric field. How might these chakra programs impact you through the related auric field?

Imagine your first chakra holds the belief that you don't deserve to make money at what you love doing. That belief will be carried into—and reflected by—the first auric field. If there is one spot for a scholarship or a team-paid position, that first chakra will broadcast the message that says *I don't deserve it*. And guess what? You won't get that financing you desire.

We'll be working with the auric fields throughout this book for a good reason: because you can sometimes make an easy shift in a field without having to do a deep dive into the related chakra. I once taught a rock climber who hardly ever reached the summit to simply "tell" his first chakra, "I'm making it." And he did! He reached the peak on his very next climb, and then he continued to work through the older issues that also were lying inside the chakra.

To make it easier for you to relate to your auric field and all its layers, see figure 3.

The Athlete's Road to Success: Frequencies

We've been discussing subtle energies and the three systems that serve as doorways through which you can access—and learn how to direct—those energies. But there is an even more fundamental understanding of subtle and physical energies than this: frequencies.

In the end, everything about athletics and coaching will come down to frequencies. This is because frequencies sit at the junction of physical and subtle energetics. They decide what will be destroyed as well as what will be created in 3D reality.

I'm going to illustrate the vitality of frequencies by sharing a story about Danny.

Danny wanted nothing more than to be a professional baseball pitcher. While playing in college, he spent his first couple of years at a junior college. (As a mom in the bleachers, I know that these are called "jucos.") He also spent summers with the same summer ball team. Among the teams they played, he was considered an excellent pitcher.

Danny then transferred to a four-year Division I school. He started out strong, but then, when he threw a few balls at the beginning of one of his outings, he felt a chill coming from the pitching coach. The next outing, he sensed the coach's negative energy coming at him right away. For the rest of those two years, if he threw a ball during one of his first pitches, he slid downhill. These types of downward spirals are common in sports. But then, when Danny returned to his summer team, he was again a superstar.

Danny really wanted to understand his school-based failure cycle, so I explained frequencies.

Between you and me, I did *not* go into the background information that I'm next going to share. And if you don't think you need all of this material, go ahead and jump to exactly what I discussed with Danny. But if you want further understanding, don't jump!

As we've already covered, frequencies are the number of cycles that an energy moves through over a certain amount of time. They are usually measured in hertz (Hz): a single occurrence of a repeating event. In other words, a frequency is a wave of energy that moves at a certain rate while carrying specific information.

Everything physical and subtle comes down to frequencies, and absolutely everything expresses on its own unique set of frequencies. The frequencies of a yeast cell are particular to that cell; those of one of your feelings are particular to that feeling. Your soul generates a unique set of frequencies; so does your brain.

You get it.

To be a really great athlete, you want to be constantly generating all the various sets of frequencies that express you at your optimum health on all levels. You also need to only "let in" or be affected by sets of frequencies that are supportive of your athletic ability. How do you nurture your best internal frequencies? The answer is complex, but basically you have to fuel yourself with the foods that will do this, exercise in the way that's right for you, think good thoughts, and so on.

How do you make sure you're only affected by surrounding frequencies that are supportive rather than destructive? Again, it's complicated. Certainly you want to be around uplifting people, work out in a beneficial environment, shop at organic stores, and more. But you can't always control what is happening inside and around you, which is why you have to have a deeper understanding of frequencies and your power to manage them.

You see, no matter how terrific your internal or others' external frequencies may be, there is a little-known aside to the tale of frequencies: once they leave your body, they return. When they reach their external destination, it's as if they reach out and grab onto the strongest external frequencies—and then they pull these back into you.

If a set of frequencies extends and gets a really cool "you can do it" message from another person, they will bring in that awesome support. Your can-do attitude will get bolstered. But if these frequencies spread out and are met with a jealous co-athlete, the "hands" on the frequency wave will close over that negativity, and down goes your performance. You probably won't even know what just happened, which will make you feel even worse about yourself.

What determines the frequencies inside us and how they best serve us or not? We're back to our discussion about programs, or the beliefs we've acquired as being true over this and other lifetimes. Some of these will enhance our athleticism—or our ability to assist an athlete—and some will be detrimental. That means that we don't only send can-do frequencies into the world. We also generate *can't-do* frequencies, which easily find their equivalent. Best case? We activate our success-oriented internal frequencies and get them paired with equally great ones outside ourselves. This is the formula for success.

Now I'm going to pick up my story about Danny again, sharing with you how I told him about frequencies. While I relate it, take a look at figure 4 and its subcomponents. I showed him a (pretty bad) sketch like this to get the message across.

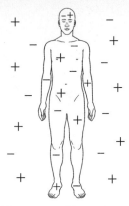

4A: There are positive and negative frequencies inside and outside us.

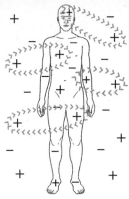

4B: We can send positive frequencies into the world and connect with positive to create success.

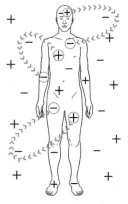

4C: We can generate positive frequencies into the world. If the external negative frequencies are really strong, the negative can be pulled in and activate the negative frequencies inside us.

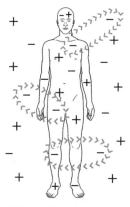

4D: We can broadcast negative frequencies into the world, and they can bring in more negative energies.

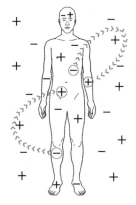

4E: Sometimes we send negative frequencies into the world, and a really strong set of positives can come in despite our negativity. This activates our positive frequencies.

Figure 4: The Model of Frequencies. Frequencies emanate from us and connect with frequencies outside us. These various images depict some of the possibilities of what might happen during that transaction. The + signs equal positive, success-creating frequencies, and the − signs equal negative, failure-causing frequencies.

Inside each of us are frequencies of success and failure. Let's call these positive and negative frequencies. There are also external frequencies, positive and negative, that can impact us. These are depicted on figure 4A.

Reality manifests when the frequencies inside us match up with those outside us. So, to get really good performance, we need to do what is shown in figure 4B and operate from our positive frequencies. Sent into the world, these then catch ahold of the positive frequencies outside us. *Voilà*—we'll be able to show up in the best way we can.

However, there are other possible scenarios.

As we see in figure 4C, we can come from our positive frequencies, which try to seek out the good stuff. But what if they only find negative frequencies? Unfortunately, that's what our seeker frequencies will then pull in. Down we slide. Then again, we might start out by sending our negative frequencies into the world. We've all had really bad physical or mental days. Of course, these will jettison into the world and latch onto negative frequencies, as shown on figure 4D. Now we're really in trouble. But once in a while, we might conduct ourselves from our internal negatives and be greeted with positive in the world. Hurrah! This can happen if a really powerful figure or group outside us really believes in us. Now the external positives could outweigh our internal negatives, as is shown in figure 4E, and it will all be okay.

Danny asked me a question at this point.

"How do we know if we're giving off positive or negative frequencies?"

We usually don't, I explained. In fact, we have about 80,000 thoughts a day, and most of these are a repeat of yesterday's thoughts. Of these, at least 80 percent are negative. Of course, we're not listening in to our own conversations, much less the chatter of the ancestors or the traumatized selves that are stuck in shock bubbles. Neither are we usually aware of the impact of uncleared forces or the chitchat of others' subtle charges that are stuck in our body.

Danny then wanted to know about the sources of external frequencies.

The truth is that there are tons of these. They can include the people and groups around us as well as subtle charges in the environment. There are also invisible beings, good and bad, which we briefly discussed in the previous chapter.

As I explained all this to Danny, I could see a light going on in his head.

He asked, "You mean, when I'm on my summer team, and when I was in juco, I could pitch really well because the coaches were so pro-me?

"Even if I threw a couple of balls, they didn't freak," he added. "They'd just say, 'You've got this.'"

He grasped this, but he didn't understand why the attitude of a single pitching coach in the D-1 school would matter so much.

I explained that once he became sensitive to that coach's opinion, he probably also started to pick up on the negatives of other people. There were pitchers from his own team vying for his spot. And how about members of the opposing teams and *their* parents and coaches? Danny suddenly started to understand why after throwing one pitch outside the strike zone, he then threw more.

Pretty soon, his pitching improved, even on the D-1 team. But he also didn't like swimming upstream. When he could, he took advantage of being a senior and moved to a D-2 team so he wouldn't have to fight all the negatives. And now, he's up for the draft.

We constantly see signs of the impact of our own negative frequencies being empowered by the negative frequencies outside us. Look at the career of Tiger Woods, pro golfer. Nothing could stop him—until he got caught womanizing. Suddenly the public turned against him. That's a *lot* of negative frequencies coming his way. Plus, we can only imagine the shame and guilt that triggered inside of him. His career nosedived, only returning once he did considerable therapy (emotional and physical) on himself.

Ultimately, freedom comes from accepting the negative within us while learning how to center ourselves in the most positive frequencies within. From there, we are faced with a choice: Will we learn how to pay attention to only the negatives coming from outside? Or can we learn how to tune in to only the positives, and better yet, become our own positive source of external support?

You'll learn how to do this in the next chapter, along with a lot of other pretty exciting activities.

EXERCISE 5: A TWO-DAY FOCUS

Select two days in a row for this exercise.

During the first day, focus on the positives inside you by thinking uplifting thoughts several times a day. However, notice only the negatives around you. Pay attention to how bad the other drivers on the road are, ways that other athletes hate you, the destructive cycles in the news. How do you feel about your athletic or coaching potential at the end of the day?

On the second day, focus only on the positives inside you, such as by giving yourself affirmations during the day. Then, deliberately pay attention only to what is healthy and positive in your external world. Notice who smiles, who leaves you room for your car when you're changing lanes, and all the happy news in the media. Then sit down and think about your athletic or coaching potential. How does your current attitude compare to yesterday's?

Quite the difference, right?

Just as your physical body is composed of organs, channels, and fields, so is your subtle body. You'll be working with all these subtle structures—the chakras, meridians and nadis, and auric fields—to make it easier to become a great athlete or athletic coach. You were also introduced to a model of frequencies that explains how important it is to be focused on the positive beliefs or frequencies inside you, as well as the positives outside you. Gaining this balance, no matter what is occurring internally or externally, is truly the key to athletic or coaching success.

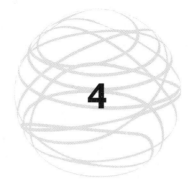

4

Get-Set Techniques:
Your Basic Energy Tool Kit

*Sports can create hope where
once there was only despair.*

—Nelson Mandela at the
2000 Laureus World Sports Awards

Congrats! You've learned a ton about energy and how it can work with you or against you when you want to excel at your sport. Now it's time to stock up on energy techniques in a serious way.

As we explore these basic practices, I want you to customize them to your own needs and goals. That customization applies to athletes and coaches of all varieties. It also applies to your everyday life, not just your expertise in sports. In fact, you'll probably find that employing this chapter's techniques in athletics will invariably alter your non-sports life in positive ways too.

For example, one young tennis player I worked with loved the sports-based practice Gamma Gameline so much that she used it when dating; the technique helped her sense whether she wanted another date. She simply reshaped the process a smidgen so it applied to that aspect of her life, not just her tennis game. An owner of a basketball team sculpted the Sports Spirit practice into a meditation he had his players recite internally. He then used the practice himself to stay patient when his kids were wired.

As a mom in the bleachers, I enjoy these practices in all arenas of life, and I want to clue you in to a fact: sports isn't only about what happens on the field or in the bleachers.

For example, I recently flew to Nashville to attend games in Bowling Green, Kentucky. My plan was to drive the roughly hour and a half Thursday night in time for games that were scheduled for Friday through Sunday. As luck would have it, blizzards and tornadoes had hit the region during the week before the games, causing wrack and ruin on the roads.

I landed on a Thursday night, only to be thwarted by a giant pothole that lay in wait between the airport and my destination—*blam!* went a tire. Pulling into a gas station at the end of an off-ramp, I was informed that no one there was available to help and it would be three hours before I could get a tow. Feeling cold and lost, I quickly used the Sports Spirit and the Streams techniques (taught in this chapter). Once I had connected with that guidance, I distinctly heard, "Hire the plowman."

Still a bit disconcerted, I tapped on the window of a man who was plowing the parking lot and explained my situation. He suggested he could put the donut spare on my car to replace the blowout, and *voilà!*—he changed the tire. While he worked, I had a great time chatting with at least five more local people who were more than happy to tell me storm stories. I even got free potato chips for dinner from the gas station, as the plowman's daughter was working there that night. Soon I was on my way again, and I exchanged my car for a different one in Bowling Green the next morning.

I've learned that just about anything is possible if you employ subtle energy practices.

Of course, you'll need a bit of faith—in yourself, guidance, and a Higher Power—to pull off some of these techniques. That's why I want you to shape-shift these practices to fit your individual needs and your faith. They're ready-made for any religion or spirituality. They'll work equally well if you're an atheist, universalist, Christian, Muslim, Hindu, or simply a believer in a "force" of goodness. In fact, I taught them once to a strongly Christian dad in the bleachers, and this is how he applied the ideas during the very same weekend I just referenced: he just called them "prayer."

He had started for Bowling Green thinking he would first vacation in Florida. But because of the weather, his plane landed at the wrong airport, leaving all the passengers stranded. (Go figure that one.) So he prayed, acknowledging his own divine self, the passengers around him, and God (his version of the Sports Spirit technique you will soon learn). As soon as he finished, one of the men near his seat signed into his rental car account and nabbed a car—becoming the only one from that plane to get one.

That gentleman drove my fellow bleacher-parent and other members of that flight to their real destination for no charge. Once there, arriving with no hotel reservation, the dad was invited to spend four days on a boat with some friends. Sure, it rained for four days and the boat never left the dock, but the housing was free! Finally, he drove on, arriving in Bowling Green right before the blizzard I ran into, where he safely hunkered down for a few days.

In the end, all he could do was laugh.

Look, the point is that life isn't perfect. But if you apply a little faith and a good attitude along with these techniques, you'll always get somewhere better than where you were. So let's begin.

Note: This chapter is organized into two main parts. The first covers subtle energy tools, and the second addresses vibrational remedies.

Subtle Energy Tools

There are a lot of really powerful tools in this section. The following five areas comprise the main concepts and techniques you'll build upon during the rest of the book. Here is a preview of these exercises.

Sports Spirit: This is a three-part exercise you'll use for everything. It can be employed as a stand-alone technique; however, I also advise you to use it before you do any other practice. You can think of it as a sort of sports prayer.

The Streams: These are universal healing energies that can help you release problems, hold your boundaries, and manifest desires.

Intuitive Tools: There are four basic intuitive styles: physical, spiritual, verbal, and visual. These can be employed separately or together for all energy work exercises. I'll share quick ways to use your intuition to perform the following sports activities:

- ▸ Gaining spiritual guidance
- ▸ Chain-lock
- ▸ Visualization
- ▸ Applied kinesiology

Gamma Gameline: An incredible process for getting into—and staying in—the flow.

Energy Analysis and Healing: A method for assessing and healing energy, such as delivering a regression or problem-solving.

Sports Spirit

This exercise is the most important to get acquainted with. That's because it enables you to engage with your highest self or spirit; the best part of others, visible and invisible; and the Higher Spirit, which you can call by any other name you wish. I think it's especially important to use the word "spirit" when undertaking sports because there truly is a spirit to sports.

I'm not talking religion, though I've already made it clear that I believe religion can fit hand in glove with sports. *Spirituality*, however, is about a connection to that which is greater. *Religion* is a path that unfolds the certainty that something greater exists. As a sports-coach mom, I believe you get to your best game by embracing that which is bigger than the everyday, as well as the spirit of your sport.

Don't believe there is a spirit to sports? Ask any athlete who has experienced that moment in which everything lines up, when there is perfect flow, and when you become bigger than yourself. You don't have to believe that Spirit is alive or conscious; it's enough to know it as a *zing* that links you to a greater force than just you.

Ready to practice the three steps involved in reaching your best self and performance—or helping another do the same? I'll explain each step in the following exercise.

EXERCISE 6: SPORTS SPIRIT

On your first time doing this exercise, I encourage you to walk through it in detail in a quiet place. I'll summarize the three steps right after this lengthier version of the practice so you can then use a shorter cheat sheet.

Affirm your own spirit. This is your divine spark or highest self. Perceive it within and around you. You might simply sense this complete and empowered version of you. Then again, an image of your essence might pop into your mind. You might even become aware of a pulse, tone, or word that can be affiliated with your true self from this point forward.

Affirm others' spirits. This step acknowledges the spirit linked with all others involved in an experience, and it also includes the ineffable spirit of your sport. If you're alone, you are inviting a bond with any invisible helpers that might attend to you. If you're focused on another person, group, or even a team, you are agreeing to connect with their spirits, not just their apparent selves. That can include becoming linked to their spiritual guides as well.

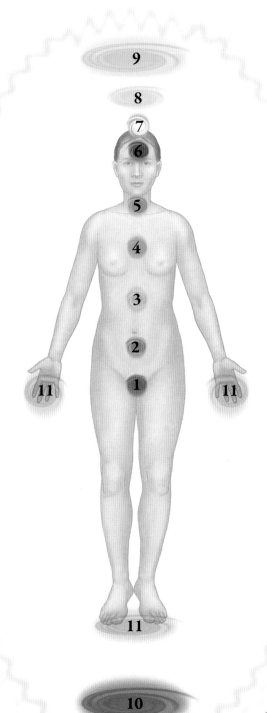

9

8

7

6

5

4

3

2

11   1   11

11

10

12

Chakra 1
(1) Red

(2) Hips

(3) Coccygeal vertebrae, adrenals

(4) Hips area, genitals, large intestine, anus, rectum

(5) Safety and security

(6) In utero to 6 months

(7) Physical empathy and manifesting

Chakra 2
(1) Orange

(2) Abdomen

(3) Sacral vertebrae and ovaries or testes

(4) Sacrum area, small intestine, sexual organs and their functions

(5) Emotions and creativity

(6) 6 months to 2½ years

(7) Feeling empathy and creativity

Chakra 3
(1) Yellow

(2) Solar plexus

(3) Thorasic vertebrae and pancreas

(4) Most digestive organs

(5) Power and self-esteem

(6) 2½ to 4½ years

(7) Cognitive empathy and administrative functions

Chakra 5
(1) Blue

(2) Throat

(3) Cervical vertebrae and thyroid

(4) All glands and body parts associated with throat, neck, jaws, teeth

(5) Expression and communication

(6) 6½ to 8½ years

(7) Clairaudience, or "clear hearing"

Chakra 6
(1) Violet

(2) Brow

(3) Higher vertebrae, pituitary gland

(4) All body parts related to eyes, seeing, overseeing, or hormones and parts of brain

(5) Self-image and goal setting

(6) 8½ to 14 years

(7) Clairvoyance, or "clear seeing"

Chakra 7
(1) White

(2) Top of head/ inside center of head

(3) Cranial area, pineal gland

(4) Brain learning centers, cranium and cranium bones

(5) Spirituality and life purpose

(6) 14 to 21 years

(7) Prophecy, or clear consciousness

Chakra 9
(1) Gold

(2) A foot over the head

(3) Diaphragm

(4) Breathing functions; holds codes to assist all parts of the body

(5) Harmony with others

(6) 28 to 35 years

(7) Ability to harmonize

Chakra 10
(1) Brown

(2) A foot under the feet

(3) Bone marrow

(4) All bone functions, genes, and epigenetics

(5) Place in the world, relationship with Nature

(6) Pre-conception, conception; also 35 to 42 years

(7) Natural empathy

Chakra 11
(1) Pink

(2) In the energy field, also around the hands and feet

(3) Connective tissue

(4) Muscles, connective tissue, collagen

(5) Connectivity with others

(6) 42 to 49 years

(7) Commanding of supernatural and natural forces

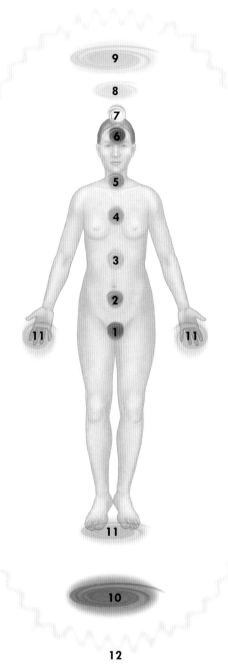

Chakra 4
(1) Green

(2) Chest

(3) Cardiac plexus and heart

(4) All organs in chest, ribs

(5) Love and relationship

(6) 4½ to 6½ years

(7) Relational empathy
and healing powers

Chakra 8
(1) Black/Silver

(2) An inch above the head

(3) Thymus

(4) Immune system

(5) Sense of self as mystical

(6) 21 to 28 years

(7) All mystical and
shamanic abilities

Chakra 12
(1) Clear or opaque

(2) Outer rim of auric
field; can also be accessed
in center of fourth chakra

(6) Chakra 12, which develops between
49 and 56 years of age, is unique to each
person and holds your own special intuitive
gifts; after age 56, the chakras begin
to recycle in seven-year blocks,
and you start over again with
the first chakra.

CHAKRA ATTRIBUTES: Each chakra can be described with specific attributes. In this illustration you will find the following factors: (1) chakra color, (2) location, (3) spinal area and/or endocrine gland, (4) primary physical functions, (5) primary psychological ideas, (6) age of development, and (7) intuitive gifts. FIGURE BY MARY ANN ZAPALAC

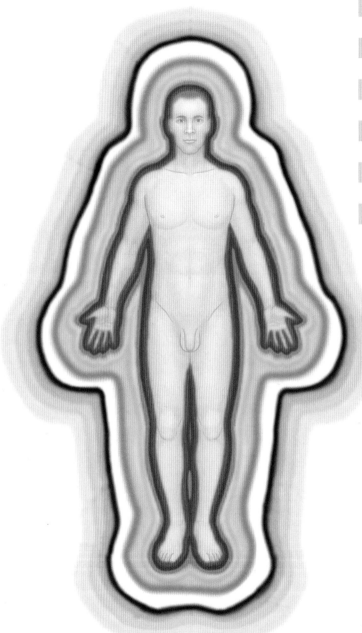

Auric Field	Color
First	Red
Tenth	Brown
Second	Orange
Third	Yellow
Fourth	Green
Fifth	Blue
Sixth	Violet
Seventh	White
Eighth	Black
Ninth	Gold
Eleventh	Pink
Twelfth	Translucent

THE TWELVE-CHAKRA AURIC FIELDS: The twelve-chakra system features twelve auric layers, each of which is affiliated with one of the chakras. While most of the layers stack upon each other in sequence, the tenth auric field actually follows the first auric field. Afterward is the second auric field, the third, and so on. The auric layers are described in order of their location and by color.   FIGURE BY MARY ANN ZAPALAC

A note on the spirit of your sport: for you, that spirit might be an actual person, such as a former player or coach, or an amalgam of the best performers in your sport over time. Then again, it could be the sum total of all the best and highest practices associated with your sport. It might even be an actual spirit.

Right now—the first time you practice this step—stop for a few minutes and sink into the spirit of your sport as you understand it. What is the sensation? What kinds of feelings, values, and energies embrace you? Does a sports figure or religious icon come into your mind? The spirit of your sport can seem animate and conscious or can be simply a philosophy and a set of principles. It's up to you.

Affirm the Higher Spirit. As I've noted, in this book I usually use the phrase "Higher Power." I want athletes and coaches of all spiritualities and walks of life to feel comfortable with defining what is the greatest power for them. I don't care if that's Humanity, Goodness, God, Jesus, Allah, Kwan Yin, or a Universal Consciousness. You can also just trust that you deserve to be attended by a presence greater than the sum total of what is known. During down times, when you can hardly keep your own feet moving or keep the flame of hope alive, know that there is a presence to carry you through and point out directions. And so, in this moment, surrender to that Higher Spirit, turning yourself over to it.

The Three Steps of Sports Spirit
—A CHEAT SHEET—
Once again, these three steps are as follows:

Affirm your own spirit.

Affirm others' spirits, seen and unseen,
including the spirit of your sport.

Affirm—and surrender to—the Higher Spirit.

The Streams

Want a one-size-fits-all healing power? Well, it exists. I actually use two terms to describe it: absolute scalar waves (ASWs) and Healing Streams of Grace. The first label explains what these energies are from a scientific point of view; the second is a more spiritually available phrase. After explaining these perspectives, I'll provide a brief example of how to connect and direct them, calling them from this point on "the streams."

First, let's discuss scalar waves.

Scalar waves are electromagnetic waves (or light) that move differently than our typical waves of light. They are known as "vectoring" rather than "transverse" waves, which means that they bend in strange ways.

The research on scalar waves is really interesting, showcasing some of their very bizarre behaviors. It seems that scalar waves can

- penetrate physical objects because they travel faster than the speed of light.
- connect visible and invisible realities.[10]
- carry information from place to place while moving super fast.[11]

If you really want to shift subtle energies, especially toward the goal of altering physical reality, why *wouldn't* you access scalar waves?

Wait a second, though. I want you to really make the streams work for you. Because of that, I have to explain that there are three actual types of light—and even of scalar waves. You'll discover that we're mainly going to use the third explained here (absolute), although I'll also introduce you to the second type (virtual) at points in part 2.

The three kinds of light? Here we go.

Polarity light: This is my term for normal light and everyday energy. Most of the energy you interact with, especially in relation to your body, is polarity light. I use the word *polarity* because it best describes its basic nature, in that every regular particle is fundamentally matched with one that is oppositely charged. For instance, an electron (negatively charged) is bonded with a positron (positively charged). I believe that 99 percent of the athletic activities you undergo are polar in nature. However, to

10   Rivera-Dugenio, "Scalar-Energy Morphogenetic Field Mechanics" and "Scalar Plasma Technology."
11   Laszlo, "An Unexplored Domain of Nonlocality."

make something great happen, you have to deal with the equal amount of resistance. That's okay if you're lifting weights but not so good if you're looking to make quick alterations.

Virtual light: Also called virtual particles, these are technically quantum fluctuations. They exist in a state called the void, unlimited potential, or the vacuum. These sorts of void-states are everywhere, even in your chakras, as you'll discover. What draws a virtual particle out of the void state? We're back to our discussion of frequencies. If you hold a desire really strongly, a similar frequency (quantum potentiality) is stirred in the vacuum. And up it rises—just for a split second. Before it falls back into the void, though, this virtual potentiality at least slightly alters the polarity or day-to-day reality. Exercise 14 in this chapter automatically accesses virtual particles, as is explained in the section "An (Optional) Explanation of Gamma Consciousness." In chapter 6, the use of exercise 26, Gamma Gameline for Mechanics, also enables the exertion of virtual light. And finally—and most directly—you can apply exercise 42, Using Virtual Light to Quicken Healing, to enhance any process you're going through.

Absolute Light: Now we're talking. This is the only known form of light in the universe that is always solidly real and does not have a twin. In other words, it can only be directed to produce what is best for everything because there is no darkness in it. I believe that the absolute light is composed of very measurable light but also spiritual qualities such as faith, hope, truth, and clarity.

Scientifically, we know that absolute light exists because it's related to dark matter, a strange substance we don't yet understand but that probably contains unknown quanta. Dark matter is everywhere around us and predates the big bang.[12] In fact, it seems to have helped create the universe and currently holds visible (polarity) matter together.[13] We also perceive this form of light in very still twists of light found in the universe and through a low hum existing everywhere, which is called cosmic background radiation.[14]

The particular type of scalar waves you'll be utilizing are made from absolute scalar waves, which are scalar waves that only reflect the absolute light. I also call these

---

12 Johns Hopkins University, "Dark Matter," and Siegel, "Science Uncovers the Origin."
13 Kettley, "Dark Matter Breakthrough."
14 Tate, "Cosmic Wave Background."

Healing Streams of Grace—or the streams—because of the definition of grace: "love that makes a difference" or "love empowered."

When they are needed and summoned, these rivers of light are constructed by the Higher Power to accomplish any aim. One particular stream might heal tennis elbow; another give you pep when you need it; another provide emotional assurance. You don't have to steer a stream of grace toward an endeavor; simply use Sports Spirit, ask for what is needed, and assume the transformational presence of these streams.

Because of their universal malleability and mobility, the streams can release attachments, gently rid us of ancestral entities, and more. They can also assure us that the energy we pull out of our own or another's chakra is safely disposed of and that the resulting empty space is appropriately filled. Streams of grace can also cleanse the energy we're moving and ensure balance.

EXERCISE 7: THE STREAMS

Want to practice using the streams? Try these steps.

Conduct Sports Spirit. Affirm your spirit and all helping spirits, along with the spirit of your sport, and the Higher Spirit.

Focus. Think of an athletic issue you'd like assistance with.

Request the streams. Ask that the streams—made only from absolute scalar waves, or grace—be delivered directly to you. They will attach wherever required, change as needed, and drop off when finished.

You can also use this step with others; for example, if you're a pitcher, you can ask for streams for the catcher. Their own spirit will decide whether it's willing to accept what is sent, so you can't override another's free will.

Close. Thank the helpers, including yourself, for enabling this process. Go about your day and see how you feel and whether additional information drops in to assist.

Intuitive Tools

Guess what? You are naturally intuitive! And you'll need to access your main intuitive gifts to perform many of the exercises in this book. For that reason, I'm going to dissect the four main types of intuition, also breaking them down into subcategories.

Two of these styles are kinesthetic, meaning they are primarily felt in the body and constitute a form of empathy. Most athletes are very comfortable with the empathic aptitudes because the body is the vehicle for sports performance. I worked with a mountain climber who trusted his bodily senses so much that rather than use his eyes to figure out where to place his hands, he let his hands move where they wanted to. A swimmer I knew always sensed where the other swimmers were in their lanes during a competition. He trusted that feeling to figure out when to push toward the end of the pool.

The other two capabilities are verbal and visual. As you would expect, verbal intuition is auditory and visual is picturesque, but you might be surprised at the various forms of these two standard intuition processes—and I'll give you a few examples soon. Of course, you can gain insights from any or all of these types of intuition.

For instance, I once worked with a slalom skier whose bones could sense what the weather would be like the following day. He'd then run Sports Spirit to double-check his assessment. He also heard psychic words that would confirm, deny, or amend his weather prediction. Then when he was skiing, he'd see images of the flags in his mind's eye a split second before they were visible and gauge his actions based on these inner pictures, not his eyes.

As I cover these intuition forms, I'll also tell you which chakras the abilities link to. As I explained in chapter 3, every chakra operates on its own band of frequencies. That makes each chakra an expert on some particular form of intuition.

Physical Intuition

Physical intuitives receive guidance or messages, or know what to do, through bodily sensations. Do you relate to any of the following?

Physical empathy (first chakra): Knowing what's occurring outside the self through taste, touch, smell, or another physical sensation. Can also know what you need to do (or not) because your body takes over and just does something.

Feeling empathy (second chakra): Relating to others' feelings as if they are your own. Also letting your own feelings determine the best course of action.

Mental empathy (third chakra): Cognitively knowing others' thoughts or beliefs as if they are your own. As well, includes following your gut sense of what to do or believe.

Relational empathy (fourth chakra): Sensing what someone else needs in order to feel lovable or good about themselves. Your heart will also help you feel what or who is good and not good for you. A lot of people with relational empathy have healing powers.

Natural empathy (tenth chakra): Sensing what is occurring in nature and with natural beings, like animals or plants. You'll need to recharge for your sport in the great outdoors, with a pet, or by doing something with an element of nature, like building a fire or swimming in a lake.

Force empathy (eleventh chakra): The ability to feel what is happening with—and to direct—natural as well as supernatural forces. For instance, you might get a chill and know that someone just directed nasty thoughts at you. You might even put in a marching order for the weather to change so you can work out—and find that it does.

Spiritual Intuition

Spiritual intuitives read or comprehend subtle energy through various forms of spiritual knowing, including the following:

Prophecy (seventh chakra): Assessing a situation as if through the heart of the Divine.

Shamanism (eighth chakra, which actually combines all the chakra gifts): Using all the mystical senses, including the other three intuitive styles, to gather or disseminate subtle energy.

The main difference between physical and spiritual intuitives is that people who are physically oriented gain all intuition through the five senses. Spiritual intuitives sense information in their bodies that originates from higher sources of consciousness.

Verbal Intuition

The verbally gifted person hears words, tones, or psychic guidance either inside their head or from outside it. They might also write, sing, or use some other auditory or musical medium to receive or share intuitive information. Hear a song on the radio that pertains to a question you're asking? Well, that's verbal intuition, which is also called clairaudience (for "clear hearing").

Visual Intuition

The visual intuitive receives and sends psychic images. These can come in the form of visions or pictures; be perceived as colors, shapes, or even slide shows; and be available through nightly dreams, daydreams, and in everyday life. Some visual psychics, also called clairvoyants or "clear seers," also get visual messages directly from the environment. Pay attention to what those license plates or billboards proclaim!

Following are four exercises that will help you access and develop your intuitive styles. I want to share a few words—okay, paragraphs—about spiritual guidance before inviting you through the necessary steps in exercise 8.

There are so many different types and realms of guides that I simply can't list them all. I will say that sometimes, the souls from living people will show up to help. Other times, the deceased will, whether they are related to you or not. Then there are sports guides, who are usually former (and quite possibly deceased) sports figures, masters, or nature beings. Even your pet might arrive in your intuitive mind to respond to a need.

I had a pretty incredible experience several years ago when Gabe was struggling in his senior year. He'd been quite sick and had undergone surgery and was then feeling like he'd never get back on top of his sports game. I was sitting in the mall having tea with my girl-friends after watching a movie, and I felt a soul half enter my body.

I could tell he was a strong Black man and deceased, and that he had played ball. That knowledge came to me through physical empathy and a vision. What he said to me was this:

"When I was in high school, I hurt my left knee. Everyone told me I was washed up, except the school janitor. He believed in me; in fact, he said, 'If you can't use your left leg, use your right one.'" I had the impression that the soul wasn't a pitcher like my son but had felt the need to assist me. I felt so moved and full of hope that I cried.

The next day, I was teaching a class at the local college and told the story. During lunch break, a student came up to me.

"Say," he said, "that was my uncle."

When I asked him how he knew, he described his uncle to me and the pain he had always complained about—in the left leg. Also, that he'd become one of the first few Black Americans to make it in baseball. During his time, he had made quite the mark. When I told Gabe about the visitation of the baseball player's soul—and the fact that a student had known who he was—Gabe was astounded. For one, it spoke to the ups and downs of athletics and the need to keep going if at all possible. Secondly, it enthused him to know that the injured man had still "made it." In fact, a few months later, Gabe went to that particular student, who did body work, for a very beneficial session.

The moral of the story is to be open to help. We all need it.

EXERCISE 8: GAINING SPIRITUAL GUIDANCE

Here are the steps to invite connection with the unseen.

Conduct Sports Spirit. Acknowledge your own essence, the spirits related to your sport, and any other helper you might require. Affirm the Higher Spirit and ask that only invisible beings that can communicate to you be filtered through that sacred level.

Focus or be open. You can either focus on a particular issue or ask to receive whatever insight you need (be open). I recommend that you hold your awareness in the inner wheel of your heart chakra. Then request that streams be sent throughout you to bring guidance to your body and chakras. Take the time needed to sense, feel, become aware of, hear, or see a response.

Engage. When you get a reaction, ask questions of any being or beings that show up. Simply pose your question and wait for insight. If you don't get anything immediately, ask that the message be given to you in another way over the next few days.

Close. When you feel complete, thank all the guides for their care and support, and return to your life.

EXERCISE 9: CHAIN-LOCK

When you make a gain, whether it's intuitive or otherwise energetic, or you just plain finally get a maneuver or idea right, lock it in! You want it to land firmly in every area of your body, mind, and soul. This short exercise will enable that.

Conduct Sports Spirit. Quickly affirm your own spirit, the helping spirits, and the Higher Spirit.

Focus. Use whatever senses are available to zero in on the accomplishment. Employ your five senses: touch, taste, smell, hearing, and seeing. Be conscious of your success. If you get a quick psychic picture, word, or empathic sensation, acknowledge it. Ignore mental chatter, and let all those awarenesses land in the inner wheel of your heart chakra (in the middle of your chest).

Ask for streams while tapping your chest. Request that the streams direct the energies of success to land in your heart chakra. Then tap your chest once with at least one finger, or imagine that this is being done for you, even while the streams spread the energetics throughout all aspects of you—top to bottom and sideways, physically and subtly.

Tap again. The second tap will finish anchoring the accomplishment.

Close. When finished, return to your life.

And when you're ready, tap again. The key is to tap again any time you want to remind yourself about what you have accomplished. All further taps will bring back what has been chain-locked. If you make improvements, next time you do your tapping, simply lock those in and the most recent success will surface at the next initial tap.

EXERCISE 10: VISUALIZATION

Visualization is one of the most commonly used athletic tools. It was actually applied to sports performance after the 1984 Olympics, when Russian researchers showed that Olympians who employed visualization techniques were positively impacted, both biologically and in terms of performance.[15] Since then, it's been described as a way of mental conditioning that stimulates parts of your brain.[16]

Visualization involves imagining the outcome of an experience in as real a way as possible. You want the body to believe that the events in the mind are actually happening. I find that visualization works best when you incorporate all four styles of intuition. Since intuition operates through the chakras, and these are body-based, you will be exercising every part of your physical self when using the following visualization exercise. Here are a few simple steps.

Conduct Sports Spirit. Acknowledge your personal spirit, the spirits of others, and the Higher Spirit. Connect to the spirit of your sport too.

Focus. What would you like to achieve? Create a statement you can ruminate on inside that has a clear and measurable outcome.

15 Ekeocha, "Effects of Visualization & Guided Imagery in Sports."
16 Cohn, "Sports Visualization."

Center in your sixth chakra. Your sixth chakra is in your brow. Send your consciousness into that area and ask that the helping spirits anchor you in the inside wheel of that chakra.

Ask for the streams. Request that the Higher Spirit send the streams from above your head and down through the middle of every chakra in your spine. These needed forces will also flow down and through your tenth chakra and to all the external chakras as well. You are now fully unified through the inner wheels of every chakra. Then ask that these streams connect the inner wheels with every part of your auric field and your physical body.

Imagine the desired outcome. In whatever way is natural for you, imagine that the wished-for future has already occurred. You are in that future. Feel how your feet and legs are operating. Notice the stillness or movement of the rest of your body. Then see through your future self's eyes. What are you aware of? Let yourself listen to noises and sounds, and request that guidance provide you a statement or an awareness that will describe why you are so successful. Also be conscious of your own essence and all the guides that are assisting you. This is real.

Conduct the chain-lock. Additional streams are now being provided to lock the future into your current body. Tap once to spread the energies of your accomplishment, then again to lock them in. If you can, keep visualizing your triumph while doing so.

Return. The guidance will now return you to the present. Bend and stretch. Reach for the stars. See how different you feel?

Close. Go back to your everyday life, and know that you can perform this maneuver as many times as you want.

Applied Kinesiology

I'm including three different ways for you to use applied kinesiology (AK) because so many people I work with in athletics are kinesthetic. AK is an incredibly powerful tool for all empaths.

Basically, AK tests your muscular strength to obtain *yes, no,* and *try again* responses from your body. If you perform Sports Spirit before using this method, which I certainly recommend you do, it can even bring through insights from your spirit.

Also called muscle testing, AK indicates whether a person, idea, activity, or even a food is healthy or not. The basic idea is that our muscles will weaken in reaction to something (or someone) that is harmful or negative. In contrast, our muscles will strengthen in response to that which is beneficial or positive.

There are three easy ways to use AK to conduct an evaluation. Following are the three styles.

EXERCISE 11:
APPLIED KINESIOLOGY WITH A PARTNER

Select a partner who thinks this practice is pretty neat. They will be the evaluator and you will be the subject of the AK. Conduct Sports Spirit within yourself or aloud. If your partner is willing to do Sports Spirit too, they can do it at the same time you do.

First, you will establish a baseline for a yes and a no. While sitting or standing, hold one arm straight out to the side. Then ask your partner to stand near that arm and make a statement that should earn a yes response. They might say aloud, "You are (your name)" or "You are XYZ years old"—anything you know is true. Now ask your partner to press down on your arm gently but firmly. If your arm loses strength, you've established that loss of strength as a yes. If it remains strong, able to resist the downward pressure, then that indicates a yes. You can also have your partner double-check by making an obvious no statement, such as by testing you using the wrong name.

In most individuals, a weak response is a no and a strong response is a yes. But you never know! Go with what happens.

Now your partner can get down to business. What do you want to find out about? How many reps to do during your workout? Which supplement might assist you or not? Be aware that the opinions of the person testing you can impact how your muscles respond; therefore, try to select a helper who has no stake in the game.

EXERCISE 12:
APPLIED KINESIOLOGY ON YOUR OWN

Need to make a quick determination on your own? There are many ways to do it. I use my hands, as I can keep my activity somewhat private that way.

Conduct Sports Spirit and then place the tips of one hand's index finger and thumb together, forming a circle. We'll call this hand A. This position is equivalent to holding out your arm.

Now create the same thumb-and-index-finger circle with your other hand: hand B. Then link the two circles together so hand A's fingers are gently clasping B's fingers and the two circles are chained together.

Make a statement, aloud or silently, that you know is true, such as I have suggested in the partnered exercise. Then try to push the circle on hand A open. For most people, this circle will resist opening, indicating muscular strength. (But you could be different, and hey, that's okay!) Now make an incorrect statement. In most cases, the formation in hand A will collapse. (Again, no big deal if you are unique.) Continue on to test for the answer you're really looking for.

In both cases of AK, if you don't get any real movement or the results are confusing, your spirit might be blocking you from accessing information this way. Maybe it's not time for you to know. Or the question might be confusing to your energetic system and you need to rephrase it. It's okay if the process doesn't work once in a while, as sometimes we just aren't supposed to have an answer to a question yet.

EXERCISE 13:
APPLIED KINESIOLOGY TO USE THE BODY'S FLOW

When my kids were young, they would sometimes ask to stay home from school, saying they didn't feel well. If they were obviously ill, like throwing up, I easily acquiesced. But sometimes it wasn't so easy to determine whether they just wanted to play hooky or they really ought to have a day off. So I would use the concept of AK and have them monitor the upward versus downward energy in their body to get a yes or a no.

The idea is that if an activity or situation is good for us, we'll feel our energy rise within our body. We'll literally feel an updraft from our feet or hips, or get a sense of excitement and "can do." If something is bad for us, our bodily energies will spiral downward. We'll lose energy, get tired, or feel low. Maybe our shoulders will slump and we'll feel more depressed.

In short, when our energy flows upward in reaction to a question or statement, we're getting a yes. If it shifts downward, we're receiving a no. If it stays the same? We're neutral.

You can test this process out right now if you want. Think of a sports activity that's on your mind. Turn it into a question or statement to be said internally or aloud, such as "I should run an extra mile today" or "Should I run an extra mile today?" Does your energy rise or fall? There is your answer. And if neutral? Well, change the question! You might find your body wants to run an extra *five* miles!

The Gamma Gameline

What's the quickest way to get into flow? To be aligned mechanically? To hold yourself in such a way that challenging emotions can shift easily and you can access your highest mental perspectives? To access your intuition to spot-on coach yourself or another? It's Gamma Gameline, a process based on achieving a gamma brain wave state throughout your entire being. The term "gameline" also loosely references you getting "aligned" with your game— and also betting on yourself, as the term "gameline" shows up in wagers.

On the bodily level, gamma is a very fast brain wave. Brain waves measure the cycles per second of the electrical impulses in the brain. The lower the number of cycles, the more apt you are to fall asleep. The faster you go, the more conscious you become.

Gamma brainwaves cycle over 32 times per second. At the highest rates, they've been associated with gurus, healers, shamans, and high levels of consciousness. I have watched clients achieve their optimum levels of awareness, healing, and manifesting when I took them from concentrating only on the gamma waves in the brain (or the brain wave) to achieving a brain state, meaning that the gamma waves cycle throughout their entire body. I then had them bring the streams down from far above their chakra system—from the very heavens—and all the way beyond their lowest chakra (the tenth, under the feet) to create a gamma-level consciousness throughout all levels of themselves: body, mind, and soul. By going through this process, you can invoke several very powerful layers of your overall consciousness. You are also able to achieve a hypnotic state without losing touch with everyday reality. You can see how the flow in regard to the energy system works in figure 5, the Gamma Gameline.

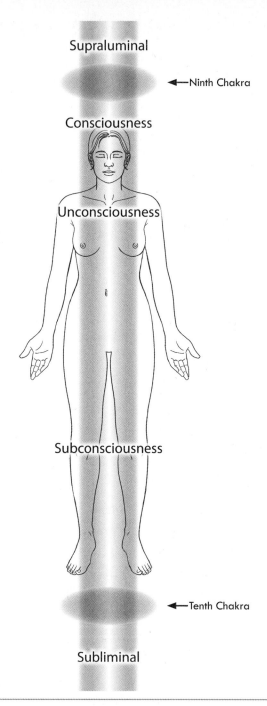

Supraluminal

◄── Ninth Chakra

Consciousness

Unconsciousness

Subconsciousness

◄── Tenth Chakra

Subliminal

Figure 5: The Gamma Gameline. The Gamma Gameline allows you to bring the streams (absolute scalar waves) vertically through your body, connecting you to the supraluminal and subluminal levels of existence through the ninth and tenth chakras respectively and the chakras oriented toward your conscious, unconscious, and subconscious.

An Explanation of Gamma Consciousness

This process enables reaching the state of enlightenment, where your will coincides with divine will. I'll cover these stages from top (way above the head) to bottom (way below the feet).

Supraluminal level. This is a place of pure grace and absolute light in which everything moves faster than the speed of light. In some Taoist philosophies, the supraluminal state is considered a "golden key" to accessing a virtual-information field that can harmonize the body with a transcended spirit. To be specific and geeky, I consider this level to contain both absolute and virtual light, so it can enable changes both tiny and huge.

Ninth chakra. This chakra holds the codes to your super-healed self. When these codes are brought into the body, they change whatever needs to be changed, and only positively.

Conscious self. The higher chakras hold the ability to achieve higher awareness in everyday life. If you're an athlete, you want the supraluminal to transform your consciousness in order to have the optimal perspective on all you do—and to allow your higher mind to run your lower mind.

Unconscious self. The middle-oriented chakras run your unconscious, or your psychological approach to life. The mental/emotional game is key to performance and the stick-to-it attitude required for great performance.

Subconscious self. The lower chakras, all the way to the grounding tenth chakra, are key to achievement, as most of our issues lie hidden at this level. These survival-oriented chakras usually run our deepest programs—and most often do this negatively. For the athlete, this means that the ways you unknowingly sabotage yourself, or invite others to do so, are secreted in this territory.

Tenth chakra. The tenth chakra assures you are grounded into the earth and linked to the cosmos. It also accesses ancestral traits. Through this exercise, you only activate and employ those traits supportive of your athletic desires.

Subluminal level. This is the space of deep stillness. I think of it as a region of the most vital spiritual truths that can completely refashion and reprogram the subconscious—and all other levels of consciousness—to the height of heights. To achieve and maintain greatness, you must access this level of development.

EXERCISE 14: GO GAMMA GAMELINE

Want to uplift your entire self—body, mind, and soul? Follow this exercise while looking at figure 5.

Conduct Sports Spirit. Affirm your spirit, all the helping spirits, and the spirit of the sport you're involved with before acknowledging the Higher Spirit.

Request and follow the streams downward. Ask that guidance send the streams downward from the supraluminal state in the heavens. Sense, see, and maybe even hear the sound of these streams as they wash downward like a water-fall, flowing through the inner wheels of the ninth chakra and all the chakras below it, as well as through the in-body chakras. These streams continue to move even lower, through the tenth chakra. From there, they gently but powerfully enter the subluminal state of deep truths.

Follow the streams upward. From below the subluminal state, streams move upward, all the way into the supraluminal in the heavens. These two streams now mix and mingle and fill all parts of you, extending beyond the outer wheels while clearing them, and into the outer bounds of your auric field.

"Do" or "be." In this gamma consciousness, you can now do anything you need to do. Ask for alignment, which will yield optimum mechanics, or for anything else. It can be equally powerful to simply allow yourself a pause point and rest in who or what you are right now. The inactivity of being can often release anxiety. Select that option when you desire peace.

Close. When you are ready, thank the guidance for all its assistance. If you desire, you can continue operating in gamma consciousness for as long as desired.

EXERCISE 15: ENERGY ANALYSIS AND HEALING

We often need to quickly—or maybe slowly—assess a situation for the energetics involved. This is a process you can use that will do everything from performing a regression—which involves looking for the historical reason for a challenge—to problem-solving. You'll even go to the next step, which is to enable healing.

Conduct Sports Spirit. Affirm your own spirit and those of others, including the spirit of your sport. Then relate to the Higher Spirit.

Focus. What's the issue you'd like to analyze or send healing energies to? Get clear on this.

Request the streams. Ask that the guidance provide streams to prepare you to seek the root cause of the challenge. These streams will simultaneously activate your intuition so you can engage with the findings.

Intuit the cause. Guidance will now bring you to the origin of the challenge. You'll actually be in the situation that was causal. You will sense and feel the surroundings; hear what is happening within and around you; see images, literal or metaphorical, about what is occurring; and be able to know through the presence of the guidance what is occurring. You might even have the sensations of touch, taste, smell, and others. You might also zero in on a chakra and find yourself anchored within it. There are many options for causal points. Here are just a few to use as a checklist.

Time Frames
- Ancestral
- Past life/lives
- In between lives
- Childhood
- Adulthood
- Chakra based:
    First (womb to 6 months)
    Second (6 months to 2½ years)
    Third (2½ to 4½ years)
    Fourth (4½ to 6½ years)
    Fifth (6½ to 8 years)
    Sixth (8 to 14 years)
    Seventh (14 to 21 years)
    Eighth (21 to 28 years)
    Ninth (28 to 35 years)
    Tenth (35 to 42 years)
    Eleventh (42 to 49 years)
    Twelve (49 to 56 years)

The chakras then recycle every seven years, starting with age 56, which locates in the first chakra.

Forces

- ► Environmental
- ► Physical
- ► Psychological
- ► Digital
- ► Missing

Pathway issues

Stuck subtle charges/others' energies

Attachments (cords, curses, energy markers)

Holds (deflection shields, miasms)

Nature of the block

Assess whether it is primarily in any one or more of these sites:

- ► Physical/body
- ► Subtle: chakras, auric fields, meridians, nadis, or overall subtle
- ► Emotional
- ► Mind: lower or higher
- ► Soul

Gain insights. Take a few minutes and ask your own spirit, helping spirits, and the Higher Spirit exactly what you need to be aware of. Perhaps you require more insights about the causes. At the least, it's vital to understand the reflections you took away from a challenging experience and how they have impacted you. No matter their complexity, all issues can be reduced to two basic bottom lines: beliefs about being separated versus connected. To understand where you land, here are two questions to reflect on:

- ► In what ways did this situation cause you to believe yourself separate from goodness and healing?
- ► How might you now repair that rift and believe yourself deserving of being connected to all sources of goodness and healing?

Ask for more streams. Request additional streams to keep providing healing and insights.

Close. Return to your life when you are ready, but also know that healing inspirations, memories, feelings, and energies will probably continue to arrive.

Now it's time to shift our focus to vibrational remedies.

Vibrational Remedies

What is a vibrational remedy? Recall that our formula for energy is information that moves or vibrates. Vibrational remedies are physical tools programmed with vibrations or frequencies that will produce a desired effect.

Cultures across time have used vibrational formulas for everything from healing to manifesting, even employing them when seeking higher guidance. I'm going to introduce you to a few of the various types of vibrational remedies you'll further apply in the chapters in part 2.

Emotional Freedom Technique—or Tapping Emotional Freedom Technique (EFT), also called "tapping" or "psychological acupressure"—utilizes the meridians discussed in chapter 3: specifically, the acupoints that serve as the portals to the meridians.

This technique has been around since the 1990s and is a support vehicle for clearing negative issues and anchoring positive beliefs. It involves touching or tapping points on the head and upper body in a certain sequence while focusing on the issue you want to alter.

There are a lot of interesting medical studies showcasing the effectiveness of EFT, especially in releasing depression and anxiety, as well as chronic pain and stress.[17] Basically, the assumption is that the tapping releases energetic blocks in order to restore balance.

Want to get into it? Let's.

17   Leonard, "A Guide to EFT Tapping."

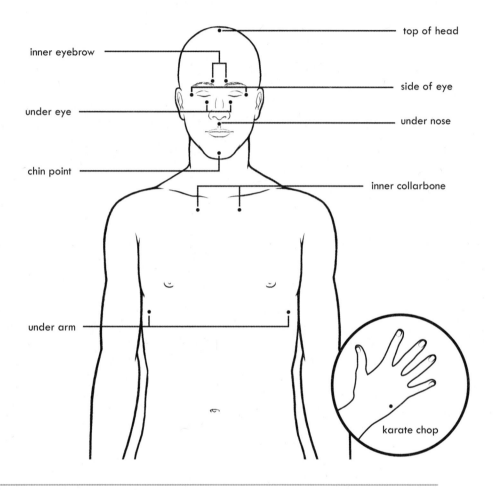

Figure 6: Emotional Freedom Technique. Emotional Freedom Technique requires tapping the shown acupoints while focusing on an issue to clear it.

EXERCISE 16: EMOTIONAL FREEDOM TECHNIQUE (EFT)

Learning to use EFT requires five formal steps and an examination of figure 6, which shows you exactly which points to tap. I'll walk you through this process while you engage an issue you'd like to shift.

Conduct Sports Spirit. Affirm your spirit, the helping spirits, and the Higher Spirit.

Identify the issue. Think about the challenge for which you'd like resolution.

Test the intensity of this issue. On a scale of 0 to 10, with 10 being awful, think about how harmful this issue has been in your life.

Create a phrase. You'll want to create a phrase that will help remind you about this issue. You are going to repeat it, internally or externally, while tapping the karate chop point, which is at the center of the fleshy part on the outside (pinky side) of your hand. This phrase must invite the acceptance of the problem, to show that you aren't resisting it. For example, you'll want to complete this statement:

"Even though I have (fill in the blank), I deeply and completely accept myself."

Tap. Now you get going with your tapping! Use two or more fingers held together at each site, tapping five times. You can tap on both sides of the body or just one. Here is your sequencing:

- ▸ Karate chop with statement
- ▸ Top of the head, right in the center
- ▸ Inner edge of the eyebrow, just above and to the side of the nose
- ▸ Side of the eye, on the bone at the outer corner
- ▸ Under the eye, about 1 inch below the pupil
- ▸ Under the nose, between the nose and upper lip
- ▸ Chin, halfway between the underside of the lower lip and the bottom of the chin
- ▸ Top of the collarbone, where the breastbone, collarbone, and first rib meet
- ▸ Under the arm, at the side of the body, about 4 inches below the armpit

Retest the intensity. On that scale of 0 to 10, check what has happened, and keep tapping until you reach zero or a place that won't budge.

Close. You're done!

Hands-On and Absentee Healing

Your hands, coupled with intention or your ability to decide what you'd like to have occur, can be your best friends whether you're an athlete or coach. The things you can do as a healer with your hands, however, are equally possible through absentee healing: the ability to send and receive subtle energies at a distance.

Hands-on healing is as old as time, often most recognizable as faith or prayer healing. It's also famous through processes like Healing Touch therapy, which teaches various ways to detect and shift subtle energies, mainly through the hands of the practitioner. Hundreds of studies have explained how the bioenergetic field—basically, your physical and subtle fields of energy combined—can impact people you focus on. As well, others can impact you through the interactive fields that compose our everyday selves.

Through the Healing Touch program, studies have verified the ability of hands-on healing to accomplish everything from relieving pain to post-traumatic stress syndrome (PTSD).[18] In particular, Reiki, a restorative Japanese healing modality—which can be used with hands or simply with intention—has made it onto the sports field.

For instance, PGA golfers have turned to Jim Weathers, a former Green Beret who has employed Reiki and other practices with players including Jack Nicklaus and Phil Mickelson. He has also worked with race car drivers, rodeo competitors, and ultimate fighters.[19]

Raven Keyes is an author and healer who has performed Reiki on members of the NFL.[20] Reiki has also hit the mainstream through its use in hospitals and has even been featured on *The Dr. Oz Show*.[21]

As I said, you don't have to work on yourself or someone else—or have someone work on you—using hands. Absentee healing has acquired a long list of supportive studies on its own. My favorite research analysis is from Dr. Daniel Benor, whose long list of books and research articles includes an assessment of sixty-one studies. His statistical evaluation reveals that absentee healing provides rich benefits, and his examination includes the effectiveness of prayer.[22]

---

18   Healing Touch Program, https://www.healingtouchresearch.com/studies.
19   Hack, "When in Pain."
20   Keyes, "Reiki in the NFL."
21   International Association of Reiki Professionals, https://blendeventdc.wixsite.com /skinergy/services2-cgaj.
22   Benor, "Distant Healing."

The truth is that Reiki, Healing Touch, and other commonly taught energetic modalities can be complicated. You often need to memorize symbols and a variety of techniques. I like to keep things simple. Because of that, I'm going to share two very simple exercises that will activate your healing powers.

Performing hands-on healing is very simple! It just requires the use of one or both hands, or instruments in the place of hands (you can use a stick or even a racket). In the process, your hands are comparable to healing "wands" through which you can sense the location and flow of energy, as well as directing that energy. In order to use your hands for these purposes, you must first figure out which is your "sending" versus "receiving" hand.

Your sending hand pours energy into others; through it, you can also share energy with yourself. Your receiving hand absorbs energy from outside yourself. Usually, your dominant hand is the sender and your recessive hand is the receiver, but for some people, the opposite is true. Both hands can send and receive, but there is typically a natural preference. So engage in the following process, and then you'll be set to perform a hands-on healing.

To figure out which hand is which, shake your hands and then take a few deep breaths. Now rub your hands together; this will activate the palms of your hands. Separate your hands about two inches from each other, palms facing, and sense the energy moving between your hands. Choose a hand and imagine yourself sending energy from that hand into the other, and evaluate that flow for intensity of sensation and ease of sending energy. Now do the opposite. You will instinctively sense which hand best directs energy and which best accepts it.

EXERCISE 17: HANDS-ON HEALING

Once you've figured out your hand movements, undertake these steps.

Conduct Sports Spirit. Acknowledge your own spirit, that of your sport and helping spirits, and the Higher Spirit.

Focus on an issue. What would you like to shift? You can select any type of issue—physical, psychological, or spiritual. (If you're working on someone else, ask them this question.)

Home into the body. Get a sense of which part of the physical or subtle anatomy relates to the issue. If you are dealing with an obvious bodily site, work directly on or over that area. If not, return to figure 2 and select a related chakra. You'll be holding your hand on or around that chakra location. Shake both hands to prepare.

Request the streams. Ask that the streams fill you in entirety, including your hands, activating each hand's abilities.

Simultaneously pull and push. With your hands over or around the area, let your receiving hand pull out the negative energy and the sending hand push in positive energy. You will sense this in your system but you won't actually direct your own personal energy or take in the unhealthy energy of another. Rather, the streams do the work for you around your hands, not through them. Tune in to whatever you intuitively sense, feel, hear, or see.

Achieve balance. When you sense that the work is done, request that additional streams remain connected to finish the work.

Close. Shake your hands again and request separation. Affirm the greater help and return to your everyday life.

EXERCISE 18: QUICK ABSENTEE HEALING

This is as easy as it gets. If you require assistance or are searching for the same for someone else, simply take a few deep breaths and conduct Sports Spirit. Then focus on the person or the issue and request that the needed streams be provided. They will be delivered, no matter the distance or the need. Thank the guidance when you're done and continue on.

Programmed Water, Crystals, Essences, and Oils

One of the easiest (and most hidable) vibrational methods is to program crystals, water, flower essences, and oils for your own purposes.

Programming involves sending subtle energies into an object or fluid in order to alter its molecular and atomic structure. In turn, those structures can enhance your own subtle and physical systems.

How is this possible?

Back in the 1990s, Japanese researcher Masaru Emoto performed a series of interesting experiments that resulted in altering the molecular structures in water. Basically, he labeled different bottles of water with varying messages on a continuum of positive to negative—think "thank you" and "I hate you." Drops of the water were then placed on slides and frozen in order to form snowflake-like crystals.

Wow! The structures in the positively programmed water? They were geometrically pleasing and beautiful. Those with the downward-driven ideas? They appeared ugly and chaotic.

Emoto proposed that a life force energy or consciousness is infused in all matter. He called this force *hado*. His theory was that consciousness and awareness can be carried in all energies, so why not the human body?

Emoto's findings have been supported by additional studies, such as one conducted at the Max Planck Institute in Mainz, Germany, in 2015. And while many people want to ignore these ideas, athletes and coaches stand at the forefront of benefiting from them.[23]

One of the explanations for these results—which can be adapted to crystals, flower essences, and oils, among other substances—is that much of our world is crystalline. For instance, there are crystal patterns in many parts of the body, including our bones. In fact, the elements that create the bone are curved and twisted, and these shapes begin on the nano, or very small, scale. The patterns repeat in what is called a "natural fractal": repetitions that occur across nature—for instance, patterns found in lightning bolts, tree branches, clouds, and snowflakes.[24] If we look at one part of a lightning bolt, the pattern appears exactly the same as the entire bolt of lightning.

---

23   Emily Hirschberg, "The Curious Study of Water Consciousness," https://emilyhirschberg.com /the-curious-study-of-water-consciousness.
24   Brogan, "The Surprising Depth of Crystal Patterns."

The theory is that crystals can convert subtle energies into physical ones.[25] That means that the subtle energies you direct into a crystalline substance can alter what is happening in the crystalline substances in the body.

Let's say you get on the mound—or in the field, in the water, or on the mountaintop—and feel defeated before you start. You can counteract that tendency by using programmable crystal substances to carry positive information throughout your system, thus supporting a desirable outcome.

There are crystalline properties in all the remedies we'll be working with in this book. You'll want to select which of the types of substances to use, and within that category, which specific substance to choose, based on the natural tendencies and molecular structures of that material. For instance, within the grouping of stones and crystals are specific types of the same. Amethyst is known for deflecting negativity. Pink rose quartz is understood as a carrier of love. You'd want to carry an amethyst if you wanted to send away others' jealous thoughts and a pink quartz if you wanted to feel deserving of a win.

For these reasons, we'll be working with the following groupings.

Programmed water: You'll learn how to program your own water—in fact, I'll give you an easy exercise in a bit to get you started—to reinforce the exact messages you'd like to receive and reflect.

Crystals: Stones can transfer information directly into your bones, connective tissue, and even endocrine glands, supporting very specific wishes. You'll learn which to use and how to use them in various chapters in part 2.

Flower essences: There are many companies that make drops out of parts of flowers, shrubs, and other plant life. These are naturally infused with the vibrations of their type, and you'll learn which ones might help specific concerns.

Oils: Essential oils, which can be delivered topically or aromatically, are each known to produce certain effects. You'll learn which to use and when.

In addition, you'll also be encouraged to use your vibrational powers to bless everything from your food to parts of your body.

---

25   Cousens, *Spiritual Nutrition*, 141–150.

EXERCISE 19: PROGRAMMING YOUR WATER

You can insert positive messages into water of any type, whether you're going to drink from a glass or a water or sports bottle. Simply follow these steps.

Conduct Sports Spirit. Affirm your personal spirit, the helping spirits, and the Higher Spirit.

Think of a message. What statement or desired effect are you seeking? Either think, state aloud, picture, or sense that outcome. If it makes sense, you can write that message on the bottom or side of a bottle, or set a glass on a piece of paper inscribed with your statement.

Request the streams. Now ask guidance, including your own spirit, to transfer the energy of that wish directly into the water. You can use your hands, as you've learned to do, or just know that your intention is good enough. Once the energy of that wish is anchored, know that the molecules and atomic structures of that water will be altered to reflect the message.

Drink. When you're ready, drink the water and give permission for the streams to carry the message into the physical self.

Gratitude. Thank the powers that be for assisting you in this way, and then carry on.

There are all sorts of techniques that the athlete or coach can use to provide performance enhancement, and you just learned several of them. A tip? Always employ Sports Spirit and the streams, and keep it easy.

Now it's time to turn the page to part 2 and apply your newly learned energetic concepts and techniques to specific sports needs.

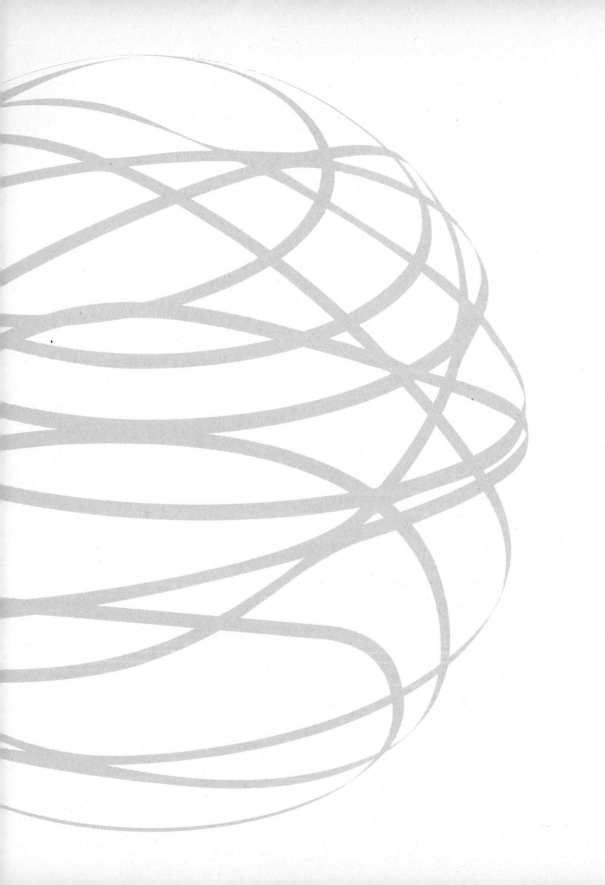

PART 2

Energy Work for the Athlete

Ready, set ... it's time to *go!*

Here is where the proverbial rubber meets the road. Part 2 is where I'm going to address the particulars of energy work as it applies exclusively to sports.

In the upcoming chapters, I'll cover the topics that speak to athletes as well as coaches (including self-coaches). Using a handy shorthand, we'll look at the p's leading to performance; in fact, we'll examine the p's that help and the p's that hurt. Then we'll dive deep into the energetics of mechanics, preparation, injury issues, game day satisfaction, and those all-too-common ups and downs—you know: the good days and the bad days.

A special chapter at the end of part 2 is chock-full of support for coaches. It contains information that will assist with both the wunderkind and the injured inner child inside each of us. If you are helping a young person, this chapter will be especially helpful. (And if you are a young person yourself, you'll want to be sure to read this chapter too.)

Turn the page, and you'll be right there with the spirit of your sport.

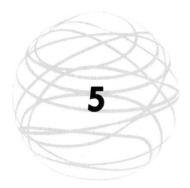

5

The P's Leading to Performance

Champions aren't made in the gym. They are
made from something they have deep inside
them—a desire, a dream, a vision.

—Muhammad Ali, World Heavyweight Champion boxer

Performance is a roller-coaster ride. Any athlete will agree with that statement, as will their coaches. You can have a great game day or workout, or maybe recover swiftly from a tough injury, only to be felled like a giant tree in the forest in the blink of an eye.

The successful athlete is able to deal with the downers and exult in the uppers with an understanding of the keys to performance—the ones that lead to hope realized.

I'm reminded of a young baseball player I knew who was treated like a washout. Following his Tommy John surgery (a reconstruction procedure named after the famed pitcher of the same name), only one college was willing to take a chance on him. But over the next four years, his performance grew increasingly better. Sure, he had his challenging innings—some were actually quite bad. But he kept plowing along, his inner spirit shining bright. And now, as I write this chapter, he's a contender for the draft.

Another young athlete I knew was a martial artist. Following an injury, even with a lot of energy work, he wasn't able to recover well enough to earn additional belts. He shifted his focus and started giving motivational speeches to youth audiences. So even there, his athletic endeavors turned into a success.

Get ready for a lot of alliteration—a lot of p's, specifically. In this short chapter, I'm going to share what I consider to be the three success p's and then the three failure p's. I'll also review these in light of subtle energies, not just practical considerations. The insights you gain in this chapter will help you apply subtle energetic techniques in the chapters that follow.

The Three Success P's of Performance

It's what you're looking for: performance. At every level of your game or activity, from the prep to the post–game day protocol. From the making of money (should that apply) to the integrity of your decisions. To be successful over the long haul, you need planning, practice, and polish.

Planning and Success

Planning is the process of thinking through what's required to achieve a goal. For an athlete, it takes a lot of tasks to get there. These can range from evaluating and adjusting your macro- and micronutrients to taking the steps necessary to enter a competition. The planning involved can be overwhelming.

Most athletes and their coaches can ensure at least the basic logistics of planning. The younger the athlete, the more important it is to include a coach—meaning at least one parental figure—in the planning stages. As a mom in the bleachers when my boys were young athletes, I can't even begin to list all the functions I carried out, from constant checking of the practice and game schedules, driving, figuring out which monies to budget for what, and purchasing of uniform apparel by specific dates. I even double-checked which kid on a team had allergies so that when it was my turn to bring snacks, they would all be safe. (But no fruit allowed. Kids didn't want fruit.)

The planning is a lot to keep up with for everyone. I remember being the summer driver for football practice as I rearranged my client schedule to be freed up for half days. The problem? The coaches changed the practice schedule nearly every day. I finally wrote to complain; it didn't help. So, the four huge boys I ferried around learned that when Ms. Dale pulled up the street in her Prius, they'd have to be perfectly silent because she was on the phone with clients. Same on the ride home. What a fiasco!

As my youngest continued to excel, there was the need to bring in advisors, paid and unpaid, to tell us how to qualify for scholarships and which showcases to show up for.

Often, I was pretty much the only mom sitting on those hot summer bleachers, as many of the boys had fathers or father figures to help out.

It wasn't hard for some of the professionals to figure out I was a little lost. When I went to visit one of the assistant baseball coaches at a nearby university about Gabe potentially playing there after high school, the coach started the conversation this way:

"So, Mom. Do you know what's going on yet?"

I admitted it was all a little over my head, and he laughed. (Now, cancel out the sexist flavor of this next comment. There really was a differential between what moms and dads did in my years of service.)

"I thought so," he grinned. "So I'll catch you up to the fathers."

A lot of kids never get very far in sports because there isn't anyone to help with the many planning stages of the younger years. And there isn't *less* planning the further up the ladder you go—there's more.

With regard to all this work, I have two tips relating to physical (practical) energy and one regarding the more subtle realms. The first is for all you athletes who don't feel like you have a good resource base. Take heart. Ask for help. Look around. Talk to your friends, coaches, mentors of all sorts. Google. Get free YouTube downloads. Join club teams, associations, or whatever group relates to your sport. There are lots of options for every sport or game. Remember to reach out to real people. There will be someone who can help. I've seen the most incredible results occur for those who are willing to be vulnerable enough to ask for help and connection.

As an example, during my Little League days, I noticed that one youngster had nobody to support him for the longest time. His parents were divorced, and his mother and stepfather, who had a daughter, were also divorced. His participation in the activities was erratic. Then his former stepfather started serving as an assistant coach, and that kid started flourishing.

The second tip is this: don't be afraid to reach way above your head. When my son Gabe was dealing with an injury, I talked to a friend who linked me up with two professional players. Within two hours, they were on the phone with me, giving advice. As one of them said, "Sports is a community. We help our own."

What are some magic bullets for planning in the subtle world? I have an insight for this area.

In general, if your undoing is a lack of planning, look for reasons you might be sabotaging yourself or setting yourself up for the same. One of my clients was a pro golfer. He was in continual financial trouble because he couldn't get his act together in the planning department. Once, he forgot to enter a competition he qualified for. Another time, he didn't have the iron he needed; he just hadn't packed it in his bag. We tracked the issue to his parents' lack of caring about his career and cleared it up through his third chakra by using the energetic analysis exercise you learned in the last chapter.

Yet another friend of mine never made a higher-level soccer team because he was never on time for practices. He's still like that and refuses to change. I wonder what inner needs he's getting met that way?

In the end, if we're failing because of lack of planning, we want to look for what needs we think we're meeting by not supporting ourselves. There is a "reason" deep inside, and we just need to uncover it.

Practice and Success

It's a grind—and you have to do it. Practice, practice, practice. Practice is the repetition of activities that allows you to meet a goal, and there are very few athletes who can be competent without it, although there are a few natural athletes who can pull it off for a while. Sooner or later, though, even those people will hit a wall.

Before I took my walk on the Camino in Spain, I practiced; yes, I practiced walking. I know that sounds stupid, because don't we walk all the time? But I had to practice hand in glove with planning. I walked miles a day in all kinds of weather, wearing the shoes I'd bring on the trip, using the backpack I'd be hauling cross country, and finding whatever hill I could to clamber up.

There is no avoiding the physical energetics of practicing. You have to figure out what routines you must set up and then keep them. If you find this difficult, problem-solve by setting up routines oriented toward your circadian rhythms: your unique times of day and night when you are energized versus ready to rest. If you aren't practicing enough or you're not productive, consider looking into the subtle associations.

One of the main inner (therefore subtle) reasons that people either over- or under-practice—and yes, you can do so much that you wear out your body—is fear. We'll be talking more about the role of fear in dealing with ups and downs, but it's an interesting feeling. Its main message is that you don't feel safe. An emotion is a feeling plus a belief, and the emotion of fear is usually linked with a belief such as unworthiness, not being deserving, believing you are not enough, or the like.

It will be imperative to figure out why you don't feel safe in practice mode, and then to heal the negative belief that is bonded with that perceived lack of security. You'll want to use exercise 15 in chapter 4 for that endeavor.

Polish for Success

After the grinding through practice comes the polishing. Polishing is the art of fine-tuning for flow. As an analogy, ruminate about what it takes to make a jewelry piece from gold. The planning stages include creating a design, making a model, purchasing just the right amount of gold, and more. In this metaphor, practicing includes making a mock-up of the model. Then we polish.

Polishing isn't just the literal polishing of the final gold piece. In order to get a finished masterpiece, we might return to other stages. We might alter the design or the model or even create a new model. Then we buff to a high level of perfection.

Notice that I'm not asserting that we're supposed to become "perfect." That's an impossibility, which is why the next section is totally about perfectionism. Rather, in sports, polishing is what helps us achieve flow in all capacities.

When we tweak, watch videos after a practice or performance, consult with a coach or guide about mechanics, use personal therapy to recover from an injury, or see a psychologist for our mental acuity, we are polishing. We are gaining the ability to get into the process of our sport in as short a time as possible and stay there for as long as possible.

From a mundane point of view, we have to figure out which polishing activities are necessary. When I was training for my el Camino walk, I made continual adjustments before the big trip, including obtaining new inserts for my shoes and altering the straps on my backpack.

Subtle polishing is more of a psychological or spiritual function than anything else. To be psychologically polished means we can bounce back when we're down and love our successes but not take them too seriously. Sports are games, after all; let's be real. If we can acknowledge the joy of sports, we'll be a lot looser when performing, and do better.

The spiritual aspect of polishing is to realize that we're working toward something more than sports performance. When we're doing the sport we love or helping another with doing it, we're actually fine-tuning our soul. Have a thing for a certain type of sport or even something else? If you're reading this book, it's because the passion of the sport invokes your inner nature. You can be something when you're rappelling down a mountain that you can't be in any other way.

Remember to return to the idea of polishing as joyous, and making adjustments will be a lot more fun.

The Three Failure P's of Performance

Perfectionism. Procrastination. Paralysis. These are the three snares for athletes, and even for coaches who are assisting an athlete. What are the energetics, both physical and subtle, of these sand traps?

Perfectionism and Performance

You want to be as perfect as possible. You want that swing, hit, throw, hook, or fly-cast to be excellent. That is a terrific goal. But you will never get to perfection, as darn close as you might cut it every so often.

Perfectionism is exactness. It's the act of being so fastidious that there can be no fault. When you're devoted to nearing a perfect standard as an athlete, you can go far. A coach can be an invaluable asset toward reaching that objective. But when you edge into fussiness, there is no pleasing you, and performance will suffer.

I like to think of the statues of Michelangelo when discussing perfectionism. He created near-perfect sculptures, but I know if we were to fine-comb his works, we'd find edges and graininess where there shouldn't be. Yet many of his statues, such as *David* and the *Pietà*, are considered perfect models of their art form. That's because he saw his job as one of freeing the innate form from the stone. Michelangelo already knew there was a figure waiting to be carved out from within a chunk of marble.

The same is true of an athlete. You are inside the body, as are your soul and mind. Your spirit knows best how to entice you forth, how to shape you into the athlete you are supposed to be. Remember my discussion in chapter 4 about the baseball player with the challenged left leg? He still became a professional player, and an amazing one. He had to work with all aspects of himself; he couldn't pick and choose.

When we're orienting toward success, we have to aim for being as close to perfect as possible, but that objective must take into account our desires, idiosyncrasies, body type, and more. We want to avoid perfectionism because when we have a down moment or day, or we don't look as good as someone else in our discipline, we can too easily spiral down. Then we'll attract negative energies and entities—and now we're *really* feeling bad.

You'll be encouraged to work through perfectionism in chapter 6 in regard to your mechanics and chapter 10 as per your possible spirals. Know that, ultimately, there is no such thing as perfection and there isn't even supposed to be. If we are here on this planet to learn and grow, we'll never quite be everything we think we ought to be.

Procrastination and Performance

It's so tempting, isn't it, to put off that morning jog? To start our nutritional plan tomorrow? There are many different everyday reasons that we procrastinate, including these:

- **Fear of failure.** That's right. You know that if you dig in, you have a chance of succeeding—but you might not. As long as you don't start, you can blame a failure on your refusal to begin, not on your performance.

- **Fear of success.** What might happen if you cross the finish line? I know that my son Gabe's biggest challenge occurred the year he was being heavily scouted. It took him the first two outings of the season to calm down enough to pitch well.

- **You don't like the tasks ahead.** Why do we put off cleaning our rooms? Because it's not fun. Neither are an awful lot of the duties of sports.

- **You have control issues.** Control issues are a matter of powerlessness. I worked with a downhill skier who would put off going out to the hill until it was nearly dark, and he couldn't ski at night. That meant he only practiced for a short amount of time every day. He felt so powerless in so many parts of his life, including his ability to get a win, that he asserted his authority in a self-sabotaging way. The causal issue underlying a control issue might include fear of failure or of success or both. It could also be a way of getting back at someone who has been controlling you. If your wrestling coach counts every bite you eat, why wouldn't you put off your fast before a meet for as long as possible?

- **Once you get started, you are scared of becoming overwhelmed.** One activity leads to another. If you start that dietary program, you know there are a lot of minuscule details you'll have to attend to.

- **Once you get started, you'll be overcome.** This situation is different from the one above—it's about getting lost in the flow. I often put off

the beginning of writing a book because once I'm in flow, it's all I think
about. I know what will happen: there goes the rest of my life.

The subtle facets of procrastination often go hand in hand with the psychological ones I've
just shared. However, I often uncover additional factors when peering into the subtle realm.

Ancestral patterns might be partly to blame. For instance, imagine that an ancestor was
warned about planting their field too early, but they did it anyway, only to lose their crop to
spring flooding. Your past lives might be influencing you as well. Say you joined the military
before you were of a legal age during a different lifetime, only to be injured or killed because
of inexperience. You'd think twice about jumping into anything. Negative forces and energies can also cause a lack of safety. Maybe the dark side doesn't want you moving ahead with
a goal—you'd be too great a source of light for others. If you're inhibited by procrastination,
maybe some of the exercises in the rest of the book can assist.

Paralysis and Performance

Then it happens. You can't. You freeze. The deer-in-the-headlights thing. There are a few
typical reasons for that uncomfortable experience called paralysis.

For one thing, your body might be unable to do the job. Maybe you've pushed too hard,
too fast. Perhaps you haven't prepared enough, and you aren't ready. Most of the time, however, performance paralysis is caused by setting unreasonable goals. You get out there and
you're not ready.

From a subtle point of view, there are many reasons we go into this deep startle state.
Sometimes we are hooking into an ancestral issue or a past life. We trigger. We've seen this
before and it didn't turn out okay. In these cases, or when we're triggering a childhood (or
even adult) experience, we're often being hijacked by a traumatized self in a shock bubble.
This isn't good, we think. *I'm going to stop right now.*

Sometimes we're taken over by a negative entity or energy, one that aims to sabotage us.
Other times we're experiencing the jealous or dark wishes of another person. Nearly always,
an intense reaction such as performance paralysis is a triggered trauma. It needs to be dealt
with in that way by doing the deep-dive it will take to find and free that self, which you can
do using exercise 15 from chapter 4.

You know you're looking for performance, and there are a few p's that lead toward success, as well as others that create challenges. In this chapter we visited the needs for planning, practice, and polish, on both the normal and subtle levels. We also discussed the problems of procrastination, perfectionism, and paralysis. The tools already presented and the ones coming up will support your success p's and minimize your failure p's.

You're now set up to fully work on mechanics. It's the ultimate key to performance, and it's covered in the next chapter.

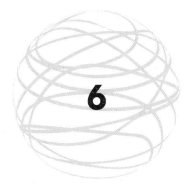

6

The Keys to Mechanics

*The reason the ball looks like it just snaps out of
his hand is every part of the body is going in the
same direction and has torqued all of the force into
the last part of the chain, the arm. Beautiful.*

—Tom House, football throwing coach,
about Tom Brady's mechanics

Tom Brady, seasoned quarterback, is known for the seamlessness of his mechanics. They line up perfectly, according to commonly accepted standards. So do the kicking skills of Carli Lloyd. But wait! She was first a famous soccer player who then went on to kick for the National Football League. A soccer player, yet her mechanics transferred over just fine.

Dirk Nowitzki, who was arguably the best-shooting tall man in basketball, is also infamous—his mechanics protocol wouldn't make the grade. Compared to other shooters, he jumped low, meaning he hardly left the ground. He also did his follow-through with his shooting hand, which is unusual, and apparently he loved offbeat drills. But he is often considered one of the top twenty in men's league history.

In the same sport, we zoom in to Lisa Leslie, the most recognized player in the WNBA and an Olympic gold medalist. When she was young, to get her mechanics as powerful as possible, she ruthlessly forced herself to become right-handed rather than left-handed and then developed an amazing high jump, jamming the ball one-handed.

Moving into the baseball world, let's talk Madison Bumgarner. Even after three World Series wins, his mechanical movements didn't change much beyond those he had learned in high school. Then there is pitcher Chris Sale, whose torqued left elbow is totally not classy, while Clayton Kershaw is known for exhibiting the best, if not close to perfect, pitching mechanics.

All these famous greats and so many more across so many sports. Some qualify as mechanical geniuses while others seem to accidentally have become amazing, so odd are their movements. The lesson we take from this is that you must have excellent mechanics your own way. Despite the fact that there is a well-developed set of mechanics recommendations for most sports, there are plenty of athletes who are successful while bending or even breaking some of these guidelines.

Because this is mainly a book about subtle energetics, I'm not going to attempt to coach you on physical mechanics. You have enough people to do that, and I'm not an expert, nor would I ever pretend to be. However, I believe that the information in this chapter can accelerate your mechanical development while assisting you with preventing the three no-no's of athletic development—perfectionism, procrastination, and paralysis. After all, if over 99 percent of an object is subtle, why wouldn't you assist your physical mechanics—which are basically the bodily activities involved in performance—through subtle means?

Lest you think you're out of the woods and you only need to perform a little subtle energy magic, I'm warning you: much of this chapter is actually going to cover the main physical factors involved in sports mechanics. After all, the subtle is linked irrevocably to the physical. For this reason, you aren't going to get out of a few lessons on classical physics. To get your body to work in a systematic way, you must understand how it works.

Without further ado, let's jump into the complicated world of sports mechanics.

What Are Sports Mechanics?

In sports, mechanics comprise the actions that lead to the execution of the sport. Sports mechanics are part of a greater study, biomechanics, which is the science that deals with a living being's biological movements. In regard to working with an athlete's movements, mechanical experts assess the internal and external biological functions of the athlete's body. Honing great and small movements and getting them to operate together is probably the most important tool for improving an athlete's technique—and therefore performance.

There are three main areas of work that most athletes focus on when improving their mechanics.

1. Correcting previously taught (or self-figured) activities that aren't working any longer. (Maybe they never did!)
2. Teaching the mechanics appropriate for the athlete. This focus requires customizing mechanics to an individual athlete's body type, musculature, temperament, and strengths and weaknesses.
3. Applying research that identifies the most effective techniques for performance. In this area, we find an ever-increasing number of tech tools and quantitative biomechanical analyses. As well, there is a growing interest in biomechanically intelligent clothing, such as the "perfect cleats" or "tech-fibered shirts."

One of the roles of good mechanics coaching—and that category certainly includes performances coaches, but I'm going to speak directly to the athlete—involves dancing in all three arenas. As a self-coaching athlete, you must simultaneously adapt teachings to your own learning style, assess for the mechanical factors currently aiding or hurting your performance, research and apply the teachings that are out there, and incorporate all the tech tools and data you can get your hands on. That's a lot to do. And it can be expensive, so you need to be smart about your efforts. Working all three areas can really enhance your preparation stage, such as when you're creating workouts, a topic we'll discuss in the next chapter. Bottom line: mechanical development is an extremely complex and ongoing process.

You'll never be absolutely perfect or seamless, not all the time. No matter what, your mechanical style will be at least slightly idiosyncratic. In the end, subtle energetics mitigates perfectionism, and that's because physics encompasses not only the ordinary but also the extraordinary.

An Initial Pitch (No Pun Intended) for Working Both Quantum and Classical Physics in Sports

I once had a dream.

Okay, I know that's not how most books initiate a serious discussion about physics. But this isn't most books, and I'm going to cover more than the types of physics that most sports books emphasize. Remember from part 1 that there are two categories of physics involved in sports: classical and quantum. My dream story integrates both the laws of the ordinary and the miraculous of the extraordinary.

In my dream, I was observing an event that was going to occur about ten years in the future. Gabe was playing handball with the man I would eventually marry. I had no idea who he was, and I wondered if I really had to wait so long to meet that amazing guy.

Gabe and my future husband were discussing events that were going to happen in my near future; I had the dream in October, and they were discussing a situation that would unfold during the upcoming months of November and December. Future Gabe was telling my future husband that his pitching was going to be lousy from November until just after the New Year. I was shown what he eventually figured out: there was a mechanical issue that was causing all Gabe's pitching problems.

As fate would have it, starting in November, his pitching really did go south—like, Antarctica south. And it was accompanied by a lot of shoulder pain. This debacle continued through Christmas, after which Gabe flew to a clinic for coaching. His pitching didn't improve, and the pain got worse. Just before he had to return to college, I flew him home to work with Shawn Kitzman, the very best mechanical pitching coach I've ever met.

During this entire horrible time period, Gabe kept asking me if my dream was accurate. Yes, if your bleacher-parent does energy work, you end up in strange conversations that are at least somewhat based on the anomalies of quantum physics. In fact, on December 31, he called and asked me if his pain and bad shoulder would for sure alleviate the next day, as my dream had indicated.

As with all intuitive insights, you are only given information on a need-to-know basis; you aren't shown every itsy-bitsy piece of data. That's because you actually have to live your life. Live it, not walk along a dotted line. In fact, very little in life is actually fated or for sure. Most events are destined, meaning you have to—and get to—create as you go, dealing with the unforeseen cards you're handed. Because of this, I had to tell my son, "The dream only said it would be after the New Year." In other words, I didn't know, so I told him to give it a few days.

When Shawn worked on Gabe on January 2 of that year, he discovered that Gabe's occiput, the bone at the top of the neck, was out of position. It had probably been out since Gabe incurred a football injury years before. That's the level of skill Shawn has: the problem he identified wasn't even in the shoulder, although it impacted the shoulder.

Shawn did a structural adjustment. Instantly, the pain alleviated, and Gabe quickly got back up to speed. Within a few days, in fact, he was pitching better and faster than ever before—with no pain at all.

Over the years, Gabe and all of the other athletes I've interacted with have benefited from my strange mix of quantum and classical physics. My premonition was obviously of the quantum variety, dealing with quantum data, which can sneak around time periods like nobody's business. Gabe's core problem lay in the bone atop the spine, which had to be fixed structurally. Why not combine the natural with the supernatural, as the exercises in this chapter will assist you in doing?

Reasons You Need Classical *and* Quantum to Achieve Your Best Mechanics

If you only go at your mechanics through the lens of classical mechanics, you'll only jump forward at the rate the body can accomplish solo. If you add in the quantum side, you can also achieve what you can consciously enable, meaning you can potentially develop faster and with more precision. That's because the exertion of physical energy alone will only alter physical energy. If you also exercise your subtle muscles, the tools of which are the stuff of thoughts, intention, focus, imagination—in sum, your consciousness—you can transform the physical environment both inside and outside yourself with faster-than-light bits of quanta, which don't stop at stop signs. They don't have to obey all of the laws of classical mechanics we'll cover in this chapter—not while they are helping you, anyway.

In other words, you can become more than you think you can be, not only what your body believes itself to be.

Consciousness glues together the classical and quantum realities. That's why the exercises in this chapter, and really in all the chapters in this book, are exercises in consciousness.

We've known for hundreds of thousands of years that consciousness can steer the body. One particularly striking example of this are the Viking berserkers, also called the wolfskins: small bands of warriors who could change their consciousness to gain extraordinary physical prowess. Their nearly unfathomable physical strength was both destructive and renowned; a battle between them and Marvel superheroes would end in a dead heat.

These dangerous warriors associated themselves with the god Odin, roughly during the time period of 800 to 1000 CE. When they attacked, they howled like dogs or wolves. They couldn't be injured and didn't feel pain—until after a battle, when they would collapse physically and emotionally. Before a fight, these warriors underwent fasting, cleansing, and perception-altering rituals to enter a trance state: a level of consciousness that allows power with, over, and through the body and even supernatural realms. Clad in bear- or wolfskins, the men embodied the spirit of their totem animals.

Evidence exists of other cultures employing consciousness-altering ceremonies and activities to invoke the same powers in their warriors. Roman writings from the first century CE describe German warriors of the same ilk, as do sixth-century records.[26] The takeaway is that it is possible to alter our bodily capabilities by shifting our consciousness.

I'm not suggesting that you distort your consciousness in order to scare everyone else off the field of your sport. Rather, I'm underscoring the point that your consciousness can—and does—shape your bodily performance.

Still don't think that consciousness, a significant talking point in quantum physics, can alter matter? I get it. You don't see many Viking berserkers on the street corners these days. So let's look at a very different culture and its consciousness techniques, the essence of which is directing subtle energies to upgrade the humdrum of classical physics.

Decades ago, Dr. Herbert Benson, one of the leaders in the contemporary discipline of mind-body medicine and a former cardiologist at Harvard Medical School, studied the thought-bending abilities of Buddhist monks on the Tibetan Plateau. He spent a month there watching the monks practice *tummo*, a meditative process, and tracked its physiological effects. He learned that under adverse conditions, the monks could deliberately alter their brain waves as well as their heart and breathing rates. They could even achieve asymmetry between brain hemispheres, lower their breathing to six or seven breaths per minute, and dry wet sheets (at 49 degrees F) in about an hour. After a while, they even emanated steam. These monks believe the reason they are able to gain control over their body is that everything is one. There is a sort of cosmic consciousness they can tap into.[27] So why can't you?

You'll learn more consciousness techniques in chapter 10, which is devoted to mental (and emotional) approaches to sports. But before you get there, I want to give you a short quantum physics lesson so you can really understand why the quantum realm can be so instructional for the classic one. My goal is to further loosen up mental rigidity to allow you to shift your mechanics without falling into perfectionism.

---

26   Hjardar, "The Truth about Viking Berserkers."
27   Mind Matter News, "Tibetan Monks Can Change Their Metabolism."

As Einstein said, matter is simply dense energy. He also called it frozen light, light being matter on the move.[28] We know that when we are operating subtly, we're actually interacting with many energies that don't have mass, and so we aren't weighed down by gravity. Scientific studies are showing that what our Buddhist monks and Viking berserkers accomplish is more than possible for us all, as subtle energies, or quanta, can be directed by consciousness—or, put another way, by intentional awareness and focus.

One of the first proofs of this wild concept was something we accidentally stumbled onto. In 2001, about three hours before and for a few hours after the horrible events of September 11 in the United States, thirty-seven different random event generators around the world became decidedly not random. The function of these generators, often referred to as "eggs," is to produce random numbers. Researchers then check these numbers to see if they become organized before or after an emotionally strong event. And during this cataclysmic event, they did—at the odds of about 1,000 to 1. The data became less random, suggesting that when millions of minds are correlated around a thought process, order can be created from chaos.[29]

You don't need to tap into millions of minds to shift your system enough to excel at your mechanics, though. Research through a foundation connected to a fascinating book, *The Intention Experiment* by Lynne McTaggart, shows that focused consciousness can alter the growth rate of plants, make seeds grow faster, change the direction in which fish swim in a bowl, purify water, reduce violence in a ghetto area, and alter the body's chemical reactions.[30] Then we have the example I covered earlier in chapter 4, the experiments chronicled in researcher Masaru Emoto's book *The Hidden Messages in Water* that demonstrated how positive thoughts made water molecules form beautiful images, while negative thoughts created ugly molecular formations.

Mystics and philosophers across time and in all cultures have always asserted that we dwell within a sea of oneness, that collective and individuated consciousness steers and dictates physical reality, and that there are multiple dimensions, and we can link with them all. One of our newest theories about time and space, in fact, is called superstring theory, which holds that there are at least ten dimensions that resonate sort of like violin strings. The Zohar, a book of Jewish mysticism about the Kabbalah, shares the same data, except

---

28   Koberlein, "How Are Energy and Matter the Same?"
29   Global Consciousness Project, "Formal Analysis September 11 2001."
30   From experiments on her website: https://lynnemctaggart.com/intention-experiments/evidence/.

it depicts the strings as letters that make the sounds and shapes that create the properties of the world. It also substitutes Sephiroth, or circles of consciousness, for the dimensions. What formulates these letters? Infinite light, or oneness, say the Kabbalists.

The Kabbalists also say that we are all capable of employing the language of creation to make and shift creation. Everything forever runs—and returns.[31] And doesn't that last phrase sound exactly like our description of frequencies? We generate and receive frequencies. We are also capable of bringing in new energies when frequencies return and sending something different into the world to instruct it in how to treat us.

In employing both classical and quantum laws to shift our mechanics, we're actually employing our spiritual birthright. But you have to practice becoming conscious of your consciousness. So do your practices—and get moving in both realms of physics with the laws of motion.

Physics and Sports Mechanics: The Laws of Motion

Newton's laws of motion are mentioned in most super-smart books about sports because isn't motion what an athlete is all about—developing and managing their mechanics, or the motions involved in their sport? In this section I'll integrate the classical and quantum laws as they pertain to motion so you can see how they interact.

Before moving forward, I want to present a couple of terms you'll need to know to make sense of the practical information included here. There are two basic types of motion we examine in sports: linear and angular. Linear motion occurs when something or someone is moving in a straight line. When you run, that forward movement is linear. Angular motion happens when the movements turn around a center point or axis. Do you have to rotate to perform your sport? Swivel your hips or head? That's going angular.

Both activities are covered under the three laws of motion, which blend beautifully with quantum lack of law.

First Law: Inertia

The point of this law is to make sure you combine linear and angular movements and mix flow with power. The law of inertia says that if something is resting, it will stay that way—and if it is moving, it will keep moving, and consistently at that. Both activities can be changed by an outside force or influence.

31   Freeman, "The Kabalah of String Theory."

One standout application of this law is that your mechanics will operate most smoothly if you're moving in the right way, at the most optimal speed, and are ready to deal with intrusions. Running a pass down the field? You caught the ball because of the alignment of the ball and your hands—your mechanics—but here come those other players rushing to stop you. (Insert whatever example fits for your sport.)

It would be all too easy for that intrusive force—who might outweigh you by seventy-five pounds—to veer you off course. That would be the law of inertia at play.

To ensure that you don't get blocked that way, you must effectively combine linear and angular movements. That takes practice and the ability to sequence the movements in your body. I cover the topic of sequencing later in this chapter, but in a nutshell, sequencing involves moving the most important segments or parts of your body in the right way and in the correct timing. Every segment must be independently operational and flow one into the other, with coordinated linear and angular movements. If you're going to stay on track when that master of defense grinds at you (again, insert equivalent in your own sport), you must generate more power than is coming at you. As you'll learn in exercise 20, you can pull power from the ground, a key in sequencing correctly. You can also employ the additional tip associated with that exercise to establish either a temporary or more permanent energetic cord, called the Vivaxis, into a specific area of land to boost your powers.

From a quantum perspective, however, you've got a few extras going for you.

You can't instantly gain weight when an opponent rushes you, which would be one of the ways to deal with the law of inertia, but you can access new data. Remember that information can travel faster than the speed of light. Brute force isn't the only way to cope with a challenge. You can also try this: get an idea, let a guide assist you, or recall something that a mentor did in a similar situation.

Remember also that frequencies can travel from inside you to outside. If you send out an SOS using intention to let those frequencies "open their hands," they bring in new frequencies. I'll show you how to accomplish this in exercise 22. Who knows what's available outside you that can pop you through a problem? Heck, you can even snare a little energy from the friend in the bleachers who is there to support you. And don't forget about the streams. They carry information faster than the speed of light while passing through objects. That means that when you are under pressure, they can activate the body segment or muscle you need and increase your power instantaneously.

Second Law: Acceleration

A lot of athletes must depend on their body to quickly accelerate or go faster, or increase velocity. Of course, sometimes you have to slow down or stop smoothly too.

Newton and his team insisted that the velocity of a body can only change—either going faster or accelerating, or going slower or decelerating—when acted upon by force that isn't already operating on that body. The shift in velocity is proportional to, and in the same direction as, the intrusive force.

Whew, that's a mouthful! Let me give you an example, returning to football.

A quarterback is running toward the end zone. Here comes a defensive player, whose objective is to drive the QB to the left, just missing the goal line. Oh, dear: the defensive player is running at exactly the correct angle to do so.

But if that defensive lineman misses a step, the force won't connect with the QB. If they are a lot weaker than the QB, they might not be able to influence the QB's trajectory. But if they hit at just the proper angle and are heavier than the QB? Goodbye, touchdown.

Another example: A tennis player hits a ball at double the force coming at her. It will go back over the net at twice the original force.

To make this knowledge work for you, you're going to have to work the major segments of your body together in sequence. (That's why the sequencing section further along in this chapter is going to be so important. It's pretty key to your mechanics.) And what's the most important set point? The part of your body that is closest to the ground.

Now let's talk quanta. Remember that quanta can jump from one state to another. They aren't like particles or individual football players; they are more like waves. While wandering, they can gather the energy you need to accelerate or decelerate, or maybe even alter the very forces that are trying to stop you. They are also always connected to anything they've ever been connected to; that's the quantum law of entanglement, just to remind you. Let's say that in a past life you were an amazing warrior—maybe a self-controlled berserker. Could you not reclaim that spirit-power and use it when you need it?

Third Law: Counterforce

This law means you can get energies outside yourself to work *for* you, not only against you. This law states that a force will automatically form another force that is exactly opposite but equal to itself. Of course, that force could support you—or not.

An example of this principle at work is a basketball player taking a shot. When they do this, they usually jump up, as we acknowledged in the beginning of this chapter. The greater the force used to push off, the higher they will go and the farther and higher the ball will go. This is especially true if the floor is stable. When you push against a solid floor—or a solid object of any sort—this will create a stronger force than if you push against a floor that is made of loose dirt or that is pockmarked. In the latter case, the flooring will absorb more of the player's force and not as much *oomph* will be generated—hence, a slower and lower ball. Think of trying to leap up when you're in a lake; there isn't enough opposing force for you to get anywhere.

You always want to max out the force you are creating. Think solidity underfoot and power from the ground up. In fact, that last phrase is especially important, as you'll learn in our upcoming discussion of sequencing: success starts with how you link with the literal ground underneath you.

<hr />

Our quantum philosophies also come into play here, as they suggest that you're an open system. You don't begin or end at your skin, so why limit what you're pushing against? Those quanta you're made of exist all over the place! If a few need to "ground" into a place far away, why not? Knowing that you're really nothing more than a collection of sound and light fields—with a little soul thrown in—is very convenient.

Even More Physics—The Details of Planes (Trains and Automobiles)

A movie came out in the 1980s called *Planes, Trains and Automobiles*. In it, just about everything that can go wrong for two travelers, played by Steve Martin and John Candy, actually does. No matter what types of transportation they try to use to get where they're going, everything falls apart.

Getting your mechanics right can feel like that. You come up with one solution, and it throws off the rest of your movements.

In order to put your mechanics together, you need to understand the various planes and forces that affect the athlete's body. I'll share both classical and subtle insights into these.

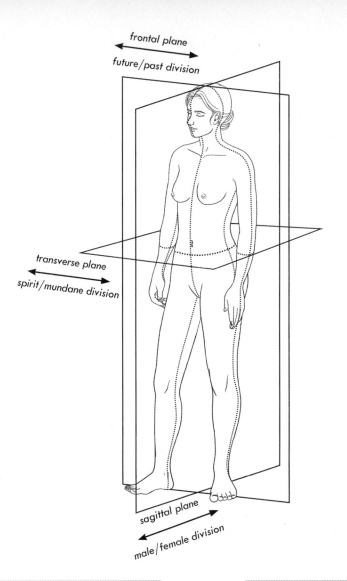

frontal plane
future/past division

transverse plane
spirit/mundane division

sagittal plane
male/female division

Figure 7: The Three Cardinal Planes of the Body. There are three cardinal planes that are vital to your athletic mechanics and performance: the sagittal divides the body into left and right halves; the frontal divides the body into front and back halves, and the transverse divides the body into top and bottom halves.

The Three Cardinal Planes of the Subtle Body. These include the male-female division (where sagittal), where the right side of the body holds our male issues and the left side reflects our female issues; future-past division (where frontal), where the front side of the body faces the future and the back side receives our history; and spirit-mundane division (where transverse), where the top half of the body holds our more spiritual chakras and the bottom half reflects our most mundane or physical chakras.

Planes and Axes of the Body

You can think of the body as a collection of planes and axes.

Your body has an assortment of interacting parallel and perpendicular planes. A *plane* is an imaginary flat surface that runs through the body. *Parallel planes* are formed of imaginary lines that don't meet; think of a three-dimensional chessboard made of two boards—you'll play on one level or another, but never both simultaneously. *Perpendicular planes* meet and form a 90-degree angle; think of two sides of a box that come together.

There are actually infinite numbers of planes related to the body, but knowing this isn't going to help you. Rather, it's vital to understand the three *cardinal planes*, as well as your *central axis* and your *cardinal axes*.

Why? Well, sports is all about motion. The trick is how to move powerfully and smoothly in order to enhance your performance or get the job done. You need the major planes working together (or sometimes as opposing forces) to produce an effect.

These bodily planes describe how the body is divided, and are as follows, including both physical and subtle aspects.

The Cardinal Planes

The cardinal planes are the three divisions of the body that meet at your center of gravity. Your center of gravity is the hypothetical point at which the combined mass of your body is concentrated. You'll be locating this center in exercise 23, and I'll also take you one step further. I'll show you how to clear and empower your center of gravity and how to unify the three cardinal planes energetically.

The important thing to understand about cardinal planes is that they are only considered "cardinal" if they divide the body into equal sections. A plane that doesn't divide an even amount of space still exists, but it is not considered a cardinal plane.

For instance, imagine that you are standing in a waist-high lake and that there is an equal amount of your body above and below the surface. That water surface marks a cardinal plane; as you'll learn, it's also a transverse plane, in that it divides your upper and lower body. You walk forward, deeper into the lake, and the water rises to your neck. The water line is still a transverse plane, but it is no longer a cardinal one. For sure, that non-cardinal plane still matters, especially if you let that plane get over the top of your head, but it's not as crucial for your actions in sports as the cardinal division is.

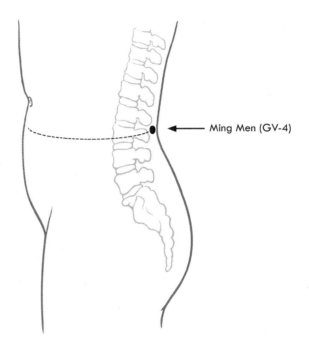

Ming Men (GV-4)

Figure 8: The Ming Men Doorway.
The Ming Men Doorway is found
between the two kidneys. From the
point of view of traditional Chinese
medicine, it is Governor's Vessel-4
(GV-4).

Your three cardinal planes and how they operate physically are as follows:

Frontal plane, physical: Also called the coronal plane, it equally divides the body into front and back halves. It's perpendicular to the ground. You're working this plane if you are raising and lowering your arms and legs.

Transverse plane, physical: Also called the axial plane or axial cross-section, it equally divides the body into top and bottom portions. It is parallel to the ground. When are you using this plane? When you're rotating, such as pulling off a spin in skating.

Sagittal plane, physical: Also called the longitudinal plane, it is perpendicular to the ground and equally divides the body into right and left sections. The mid-sagittal or median plane goes through the midline structures, and other sagittal planes are parallel to it. You're working this plane when you're kicking a football, walking, or squatting. These planes—from a physical perspective—are illustrated in figure 7. Then let's take a look at these three cardinal planes from a subtle point of view, also illustrated in figure 7.

Frontal plane, subtle: The front of the body and the front sides of the chakras face the future. Issues that inhibit the effectiveness of any frontal plane, but especially the cardinal one, suggest a fear or anxiety about the future, or the sense that your dreams aren't going to happen. You might also be unclear about what is going to transpire, how to design or act upon your wishes, or even what to want.

The back of the body and the back sides of the chakras face the past and receive historical data. That includes information from this life, past lives, and your soul. It also has the potential to receive amazing spiritual qualities that can greatly empower your athleticism.

Transverse plane, subtle: In general, the lower part of the body, and the chakras associated with it, are about your everyday and physical reality. The bottom part of your physical self links to the earth and is dependent on your grounding. If something is off below the heart, you're dealing with ancestral, primal, emotional, or mental challenges or dysfunctions, and you have to build again from the ground or lineage up. There is a singular place to work with these types of issues, which is covered in exercise 24; figure 8 depicts the Ming Men Doorway.

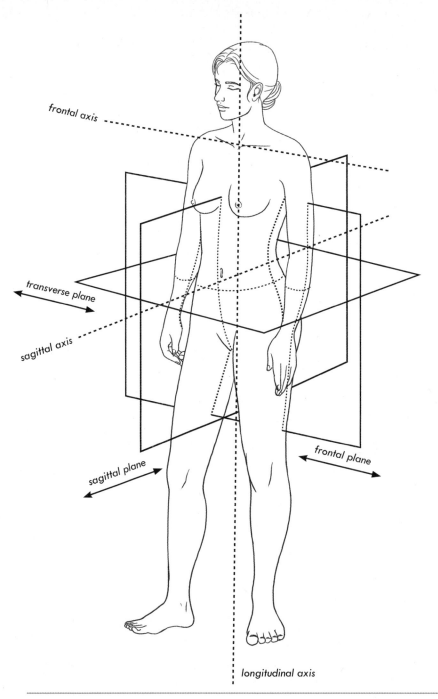

Figure 9: The Three Axes of Movement (and the Three Intersecting Cardinal Planes).
There are three main axes of movement known to athletes. In this illustration you can see how each axis relates to a cardinal plane.

The higher part of the body, from the heart up, is more spiritually inclined. Issues in getting this bodily area to work well will focus on your perceptions about relationships, spiritual guidance, your higher intuitive faculties, and your belief that you deserve to master power.

Sagittal plane, subtle: In most energy systems, the right side of the body relates to issues with your own male aspects, with your father, with men, and with masculinity. The left side holds and reflects ideas about your female traits, your mother, women, and femininity. We all have both parts.

Exercise 25 is devoted to clearing and strengthening all three cardinal planes of the body via the subtle cardinal planes.

The Axes

An axis is a straight line along which an object rotates. Movements at joints happen around an axis, but so does motion in regard to planes and any moveable segment of the body. In fact, an axis is also defined as an imaginary line at right angles to a plane.

For our purposes, there are three main axes you need to understand. I'll describe them along with a few terms related to the planes and axes that will pop into your life if you're taking your sport seriously.[32]

Frontal Mediolateral Axis (Also Known as the Mediolateral or Transverse Axis): Mediolateral means that we take our imaginary pin and insert it from a lateral (side) approach. This axis projects from the medial side of the joint and extends out the lateral side. The position of the pin allows only forward and backward movement (flexion and extension) in the sagittal plane about this axis.

In the limbs, flexion decreases the angle between the bones (bending of the joint), while extension increases the angle and straightens the joint. For the upper limb, all anterior-going motions are flexion and all posterior-going motions are extension.

Sagittal Axis (Also Known as the Anterior-Posterior or Anteroposterior Axis): Imagine a pin that inserts through a joint from front to back (anteriorly and posteriorly), effectively pinning down the joint to limit its potential freedom of

---

32   Edwards, "Axis of Rotation," and University of Adelaide, "Types of Body Movements."

motion. For example, you can think of a pin entering through the front of the hip joint and exiting out the back. Because of the pin's position, the only movement allowed about this axis is lateral movement (abduction or adduction) in the frontal plane.

Abduction moves the limb laterally away from the midline of the body, while adduction is the opposing movement that brings the limb toward the body or across the midline.

Longitudinal Axis: This is the vertical axis that runs up and down through the spine and is formed from the intersection of the sagittal and frontal planes. When you're skating in a spin, you are rotating around this axis. Same with swinging a baseball bat or golf club. I also call this axis the gamma axis to relate to the spine in the subtle as well as physical dimensions.

I introduced the nadis in chapter 3, and you'll learn more about them in chapter 9, at which point you'll be able to see the three main nadis in figure 10. In a nutshell, the spine is the sushumna nadi, and it subdivides into three tubes nested one inside the other on the subtle level. You can accomplish almost all of your mechanical corrections on the subtle level by going into gamma consciousness. In exercise 26 I'll have you practice this while in active motion performing your sport; you'll also be adapting it to ideas I'm going to introduce in the next few sections of this chapter.

Additional Movement Terms

There are a few other terms that can be helpful for the sports-minded individual. (Exercises in this book address a few of these concepts.) They are as follows, seen from both a physical and subtle point of view:

Force. Physically, a force is a push-and-pull action that can alter the state of rest or movement. On a physical level, you want all forces to go toward your intended direction. Subtly, as we discussed in chapter 2, a force is a field of energy impacting us that can also carry subtle charges or energies. You want to clear all harmful forces (or their entrance and exit points and pathways) and negative subtle charges. Doing so frees up your physical forces to work unimpeded. Use exercise 15 to help you do exactly that in relation to your mechanics.

Friction. This is the force that occurs when one body moves across the surface of another; it always opposes the forces that create the motion. In the subtle realm, friction exists where there are two contrary forces—or even emotions or ideas—causing us to choose between them or engage in some sort of peacemaking.

Gravity. The force that attracts anything that has mass to the center of the earth. On the subtle level, quanta are not controlled by gravity, as they have no mass or weight. They can be freely accessed and used.

"Center of gravity" is described in the next section about sequencing and covered in exercise 23. The importance of this place is that if it shifts, you become destabilized and need to stabilize again.

Momentum. Mass times velocity. The movement of a body (say, a ball) increases if it collides with another body (like a bat). On a subtle level, you can create increased momentum by activating subtle energies that can in turn force more power into your muscles and other body parts. Exercise 27 can help you do this.

Stability. This is your objective when you want to control or balance the mass of your body as you're moving or getting ready to move. You need to restabilize if an activity (or a thought, feeling, or external force) shifts your center of gravity.

Velocity. The measure of a body's motion in a particular direction. In the subtle world, you can use subtle energies to focus and zero in on the types of motion and direction you are seeking. Try exercise 27 for this too.

Sequencing: Mastering Your Mechanics

As I briefly shared, sequencing is the coordination of parts or segments of the body. In the subtle world, you can use subtle energies to synchronize either your body segments or your subtle energy structures; I'll show you how to do both in exercise 28. As we'll briefly discuss in the next chapter, you can also sequence your workouts so you get the most out of them.

In terms of mechanics, sequencing is the key to mastery. I'll next describe two important forms of sequencing—the kinetic chain and kinematics—from a physical standpoint, as well as a few of the subtle structures involved.

The Kinetic Chain

Kinetics is the action of forces that produce or change motion. The kinetic chain refers to the mechanical system by which athletes accomplish the tasks needed to function in a sport. Movements must impact a set of body parts correctly and in a coordinated way for proper and powerful performance. Picture this chain of motions as a set of hinges or links that allow smooth operation from the bottom to the top of the body, whether these hinges are joints or segments of vertebrae. These interconnected segments, which number five in most systems, produce force through pushing or pulling efforts. If there is a problem in one hinge, it will throw off the next, and so on.

There is a consistent kinetic chain that applies to most sports, although you'll want to learn the specific hinges in the chain for your own sport. In my research I have found descriptions of two different flows of motion. One is as follows and is inclusive of joints and sections of vertebrae, as well as the chakras found closest to these spots.

- Ankle joints (tenth chakra)
- Knee joints (tenth chakra)
- Hip joints (first chakra)
- Lumbar spine (low back—coordinates first, second, and third chakras)
- Thoracic spine (mid-back—fourth chakra)
- Cervical spine (neck—fifth chakra; upward flow reaches to sixth, seventh, eighth, ninth, and eleventh chakras)

The other description of the kinetic chain checkpoints, which is more joint based, is as follows; it is also described with the chakra affiliations.

- Feet and ankles (tenth chakra)
- Knees (tenth chakra)
- Hip and pelvis (mainly first and second chakras; inclusive of third in a secondary fashion)
- Shoulders (fourth and fifth)
- Head (sixth and seventh; reaches upward and around into eighth, ninth, and tenth chakras)

There isn't much difference between the systems because these descriptions make the same ultimate point: you need to have flow in movements to create flow when performing. Otherwise, down goes your performance and you are more prone to injury. However, when running through exercise 28, you might find you prefer one chain to another, even if it's only in the subtle energetic phase.

Most athletes work each chain with a specific set of exercises designed to strengthen that area, and then work sub-regions together, until finally putting the entire sequence into a single flow. As I'll explain in the next chapter, you'll want to research your own sport to discover which open versus closed exercises you should do for each link in the chain. Fundamentally, however, there are two types of physically based kinetic exercises. An open chain-link exercise is one in which the terminal or ending joint in the chain can move. A closed-link exercise is distinguished by the opposite—that ending joint remains stationary.

Kinematics

Kinematics is the mechanics of motion. Unlike the study of kinetics, the study of kinematics doesn't deal with forces; rather, it's a geometrical point of view, so it deals with the displacement and velocity of the body's various joints and segments. Its study is also conducted in the area of biomechanics.

For example, in golf kinematics will focus on the motion of the swing: the shape of the club's path, the positions of your body and the club during your swinging movements, and the ways you speed up or slow down to get the best impact. A lot of the analysis here involves looking at how your center of mass moves in a linear way while you're doing an activity, as well as the angular movements of the body around your center of mass. If you believe you'll benefit from working with kinematics, I've included an exercise in this chapter that draws on geometric figures and their meanings. You can use this same process, exercise 29, to support your kinetic chain.

The following exercises have been referred to in the body of this chapter, and when possible I have introduced them in the order in which they appear.

EXERCISE 20:
GROUNDING FOR PULLING IN AND PUSHING OFF

There are two reasons to perform grounding:

- ▸ to pull needed elemental (earthly) energies into yourself
- ▸ to fill a surface area with strong subtle energies so you can easily push off of it

Pulling energies into your system is a useful way to strengthen your kinetic chain and fill yourself with subtle power. It will also help you maintain your center of gravity, so that part of this grounding technique will also show up in the related exercise 23, Stabilizing Your Center of Gravity.

As for empowering a "grounding" surface: earlier in this chapter we discussed the fact that good mechanics often relies on your ability to push off a strong surface. Often that's the ground, whether it's made of dirt, grass, turf, concrete, or what have you, but perhaps it's ice. Maybe you're in the Special Olympics and you push off metal, or you're a gymnast and must create force against the balance beam or parallel bars. How about those swimmers? Sure, they push off the edge, but they also have to find a way to transform the water into a grounding mechanism. No matter what, the following exercise will help you build a subtle energetic ground; the add-on tip will help you use a special energy body called the Vivaxis to temporarily or permanently send a grounding cord into a specific area of land.

Start by doing Sports Spirit and then enter Gamma Gameline, which you were taught to use in chapter 4. Practice this technique so it's instantaneous. You now have vertical flow, which will also engage your kinetic chain. Ask that the upcoming flow of the streams from the subluminal level of energy be filled with any elemental energies your body needs to strengthen your bond to the center of the earth. Through this up-flowing energy, you'll receive all the elements—described in "Your Essential Elements" on page 134—you need to be filled with power.

Next, request that these same upward streams fill the surface you consider your "ground" with all the strengthening elements. These subtle elements can fill in holes or compensate for any weak surfaces.

Once you've established this two-purpose flow, request that guidance keep it going for as long as needed.

EXERCISE 21:
ESTABLISH A VIVAXIS GROUNDING BRANCH

Do you feel like the environment often throws you off? Are your mechanics often slippery because you really can't get your feet under you or manage a vital part of your kinetic chain? Then you need to establish a Vivaxis root in a region of land that supports your mechanics.

The Vivaxis is an energy body that is activated at birth and that originally bonds us to the surrounding land or natural terrain. It emanates from the navel, and it remains connected to that land throughout our life so we have a two-way flow of natural energies between us and our original environment.

But life doesn't always work out as planned.

Sometimes the Vivaxis fails to be established, and an unestablished Vivaxis can make it hard for us to create a springy force when we're operating in our sport; that's one way this force can be problematic. Or it might be anchored in a site where we lived during a past life. It could be locked into ancestral land or even another planet. Unhealthy energies embedded in the source point of our Vivaxis can sometimes leach into us and cause physical or emotional disturbances. To address these difficulties and boost your sportiness—and actually all aspects of your life—this exercise tip will help you find and cleanse your Vivaxis, plant or replant it, and then activate it.

The Vivaxis can branch, which means its roots can be located at many sites. You can also intentionally anchor the roots in many areas, so keep that in mind as you walk through these steps.

Conduct Sports Spirit. Affirm your spirit, the spirits surrounding you, the spirit of your sport, and the Higher Spirit.

Request intuitive insight. Ask that guidance help you intuitively hear about, see, feel, or otherwise perceive the current state of your Vivaxis. Is it planted? Where? Is that relationship suiting you? Has it perhaps failed to be embedded? Remain in this step until you have a sense of how the energy entering and being released through a current Vivaxis root is either supporting or harming you.

Ask for stronger planting or replant. Now allow guidance to deepen your current Vivaxis root, if it is a positive one, while cleansing and renewing it. If a new root or re-rooting is required, ask to be shown where the root or roots are going.

Activate. Now turn it on! Guidance fully awakens and activates your root or roots, which are even now being filled with all the natural elements and energies you require. Everything you're ready to release is washed out through your Vivaxis.

Release yourself. When you feel finished, ask to be released from this process. Know that you can rewire your Vivaxis if need be.

Your Essential Elements

There are just twelve subtle elements that construct all of natural and supernatural reality. I will reference these in many chapters from this point on. Here I'll describe each element and the types of energies it provides.

Element	Qualities
Fire	Passion, purification, physical power; energizes
Water	Intuitive flow, emotional cleansing
Air	Shares and releases ideas
Earth	Builds, fortifies, strengthens, protects
Metal	Deflects negativity, allows transmission of higher messages
Stone	Holds and communicates history; a "rock" upon which you stand for solidity
Wood	Buoys, cheers, invites adaptability
Ether	Transmits higher consciousness; gives you a "God mind"
Star	A combination of fire and ether; represents burning passion or purpose
Light	All types and colors of light deliver love
Sound	All types and tones of sound increase power
Presence	The energy of the Higher Spirit; allows you to be your own "I Am"

EXERCISE 22: ADDING NEW FREQUENCIES

The phrase already shared in this chapter about our energetic connection to the universe is so compelling. Remember it? "Everything forever runs—and returns." We are constantly "running" frequencies into the world and bringing back matching or new ones. Recognizing the power of this natural flow, here's a short exercise that will help you send out frequencies attuned to an intention so you can bring back positive frequencies that will level up your mechanics.

After conducting Sports Spirit, create a desire about your mechanics (or any other need, for that matter) in the middle wheel of your heart chakra. That desire constitutes your intention. You might feel or sense it, see it, or even compose a statement about it.

Then, on your next out-breath, request that the streams carry that intention into the world via your physical heart's electromagnetic field, which is hundreds of times stronger than any other bodily field. Simultaneously, this intention is sent via the streams through your entire auric field, moving beyond the twelfth and most external auric layer. On the next in-breath, the streams return into you a set of frequencies attuned to your intention. They are shared throughout your system to assist your mechanics, physically and subtly.

EXERCISE 23: STABILIZING YOUR CENTER OF GRAVITY

Your center of gravity is the balance point in your body. Looking at it as a plane, it's exactly in the center of your three cardinal planes. Physically, it's often found right around the belly button.

In many sports, having a low, strong center of gravity is often the key to success—especially in contact sports. Extreme pressure, physical or emotional, can knock you out of your center of gravity. That can throw off your sequencing, balance, and even your thoughts.

There are a lot of physical activities that can strengthen the actual physicality of your center of gravity, including those that work on your legs and core stabilizer muscles. But what can you do subtly?

In energy work, we often talk about an "energetic center." This is usually the chakra that contains our consciousness, in which our soul dwells the most often. That chakra is frequently the heart chakra, but it can actually be any chakra or even an auric field.

Obviously, if your subtle center is in a different spot from your physical center of gravity, that's not useful—unless you learn how to (a) temporarily move your subtle center or (b) connect your subtle center to your center of gravity. Either of these actions can serve to empower your physical center of gravity and even help you stabilize it should you get thrown off. We'll be walking through the following steps to accomplish these important goals:

- ► Locate your physical center of gravity.
- ► Find your current subtle chakra that serves as your subtle center.
- ► Learn how to move or connect your subtle energy center to your physical center of gravity.

Conduct Sports Spirit. Affirm your spirit, the helping spirits, the spirit of your sport, and the Higher Spirit.

Ask for the streams. Request that the streams be provided for this process.

Locate your physical center of gravity. Take a few deep breaths and request that guidance assist you with finding your best-case center of gravity. You'll have a feeling of it—maybe a pressure in a part of your body. Perhaps you'll picture it or even hear an intuitive voice naming that spot. You could even think backward in time to find it by remembering a time when you were exceptionally strong and balanced while performing. Where was that stable area? That's your physical center of gravity.

Find your subtle center. Where does your soul mainly hang out? What chakra pops into your mind when you search for your subtle center? You'll sense an equal amount of subtle energy above and below it and feel it as the most enlightened and vital of the chakras. Hang out in the inner wheel of this chakra.

Perform the shifting you need. See if you feel comfortable shifting your subtle center energy into the physical center of gravity. Sense the streams carrying the energy from that chakra into your physical center, and then get a sense of whether that is comfortable for you. If so, know that you can perform this maneuver temporarily to improve your mechanics on an as-needed basis.

If that does not fit for you, simply ask the streams to link your physical center of gravity with your subtle center chakra through the inner wheels of the chakras in both areas. Feel the energy flowing between these areas and how potent and strong you feel. This technique then might qualify as a means for stabilizing your physical center of gravity and improving your mechanics as needed.

Close. Affirm the assistance of the guidance and close off when you're ready. You can use this exercise anytime.

EXERCISE 24: THROUGH THE MING MEN DOORWAY

The Ming Men Doorway is a subtle portal that is activated before conception. Lying between the two kidneys, it receives ancestral energies that will impact you—positively and negatively—throughout your life. It is also found on the fourth point of the Governor Vessel meridian in traditional Chinese medicine, a yang (male) meridian.

These ancestral energies are powerful. For one thing, they program your epigenome, which sets you up for repetitive ancestral triggering as well as for good luck and good fortune. And think of it: there are a lot of negative experiences in your ancestral bed, including attachments and holds you may have inherited. That's why you should especially clear out this doorway if your mechanics are impacted by the lower chakras, such as the tenth chakra (involves grounding, inherited, and bone issues), first chakra (physical, monetary, strong fears), second chakra (your own and others' emotions and lack of creative problem-solving), and third chakra (inability to establish structure, being impacted by your own and others' negative beliefs). Also work this point if the lower part of a transverse plane or axis is off, if the lower parts of the kinetic sequences aren't aligned (those related to the tenth, first, second, or third chakras), or if you believe you have inherited attachments or holds.

Conduct Sports Spirit. Acknowledge your own spirit, the helping spirits, the spirit of your sport, and the Higher Spirit.

Center in the Ming Men Doorway. See figure 9 to locate the Ming Men Doorway on the back of your body. To center there, you can either touch that point or request that guidance locate you in the middle of this acupoint.

Focus on the issue(s). Calmly think about the challenge(s) you are having. How do they seem to involve you physically? How do they affect your mechanics? Feel any feelings you have about these issues, but know that your focus will be solution based.

Receive intuitive guidance. Allow all your intuitive insights to be activated. Now allow these faculties to instruct you about the issues underneath your challenge(s). What chakra(s) might be involved? In what ways? What might be the origin of any obvious problems? How is your ancestral lineage involved? Are there any attachments or holds? Remain open to receiving insight in regard to these and all other causal issues. You can return to this part of the exercise if you need to spend more time with this process.

Request the streams. It's time to allow guidance to send the streams into the Ming Men Doorway from the back. Often, the most powerful way to allow change is to request that the Higher Spirit divide into two major spiritual forms: the Divine Mother and the Divine Father. In this way, everything negative that you've inherited from Mom and Dad (and all sides of the family) is replaced by influences from "perfect parents." Know that you're being freed of negative programs, including energetic constructs, even as positive ones are enhanced. New ideas that would benefit you are activated as well.

Return. Remain in this process for as long as you can feel the energy moving, and then return to your life when you are ready.

I suggest that you practice this exercise during low-pressure times so you can perform it quickly when you are actually in game day.

EXERCISE 25: CLEARING AND STRENGTHENING THE THREE CARDINAL PLANES OF THE SUBTLE BODY

Of course you'll want to strengthen the three cardinal planes of the physical body by doing physical exercises and techniques. But there is a lot you can do to support these efforts energetically.

As a reminder, the three physical planes relate to the three subtle planes in these ways:

Physical	*Subtle*
Sagittal—right & left sides	Male-female—right & left sides
Frontal—front & back sides	Future-past—front & back sides
Transverse—top & bottom	Spirit-mundane—top & bottom chakras

I'm going to walk you through the balancing of all three of these planes independently and then allow you to integrate them all. Be aware, however, that at any point you can simply conduct Sports Spirit, request the streams, and work with a single plane that is indicated in your mechanical difficulties.

After conducting Sports Spirit, request the streams. Then walk through these four steps, each devoted to a specific subtle plane.

Male-female healing. The right side of the body relates to issues involving men, male energy, or masculinity. These often show up as physical challenges and weaknesses, an inability to accomplish physical or everyday goals, or difficulties accomplishing an aspect of mechanics. The left side pertains to energies involving women, female energy, or femininity. These problems are often revealed as emotional and motivational in nature. The following steps will assist you in addressing all of these.

> 1: Figure out which side is involved. Is the physically oriented sagittal issue mainly occurring on the right or left side, or both? Zoom in and then request to intuitively clarify the cause of that challenge. Where did it originate? With whom or what? Are there attachments, holds, or entities? How are you being affected? Remain in this question-asking place until you are satisfied.

> 2: If pertinent, access a chakra. Is the actual pain or challenge related to a specific chakra? You can always work with the chakra that is located near the problem.

> 3: Allow cleansing and transformation. Request that the streams release you from issues that have settled in both the physical and subtle tissues. Allow an activation of healthy energies in the inner wheel of any chakra(s) that pertain, and then allow a complete rebalance. Close when finished.

Future-past healing. Issues in the front part of our frontal plane relate to the future. Maybe we're scared of what the future holds. Perhaps we doubt our athletic success or that our mechanics will ever come together—or that if they do, they will hold together. Maybe the future seems cloudy. Whatever the case, if our soul is too far forward in relation to the center of a chakra or the spine in general, we'll experience energetic anxiety. We are literally over-scanning the future for potential problems.

If a problem is held in the back side of our frontal plane, we're holding on to a historical issue, whether it is our own from this lifetime or another lifetime or an ancestor's issue. Perhaps we think that history will repeat itself: *Yup, the last time I got my mechanics right, I slid downhill again.* And maybe you will, but history doesn't actually repeat itself! Every second is fresh and new. You'll experience rear frontal plane challenges in a part of the body or chakra area that just can't let go, which also means that your soul is too far back in relation to a chakra or to the spine, causing energetic depression. If that's the case, try these steps.

1: Figure out which side is involved. Is the physically oriented frontal plane issue mainly affecting your front or back side or both? Ask for guidance to relay the cause of that challenge. Where did it originate? With whom or what? Are there attachments, holds, or entities? How are you being affected? Remain in this question-asking place until you are satisfied.

2: If pertinent, access a chakra. Is the pain or problem associated with a specific chakra? You can always work with the chakra that is located nearest the problem.

3: Allow cleansing and transformation. Request that the streams release you from issues that have settled in both the physical and subtle tissues. Allow an activation of healthy energies in the inner wheel of any chakra(s) that pertain, and then allow a complete rebalance. Commit to remaining located in the present, in the here and now. If you slip, use Gamma Gameline as needed to hold you in the moment. Close when finished.

Spirit-mundane healing. From the mid-level of the heart chakra upward, you mainly process spiritually oriented issues. These deal with your conscious reality and also your sense of wholeness and destiny. The chakras found below the mid-level of the heart chakra are quite dense. That doesn't mean they are stupid; rather, they will have an extensive effect on you: physically, emotionally, and mentally. Often they create positives and negatives in the physical tissue. Provide transformation through these steps.

1: Figure out which side is involved. Spiritually oriented transverse issues show up in the top half of the body. Physically based ones appear in the bottom half of the body. Of course, you can experience a midline challenge, in which case you're dealing with both types of concerns. Take a deep dive and let your intuition show you the cause of that challenge. Where did it originate? With whom or what? Are there attachments, holds, or entities? How are you being affected? Remain in this question-asking place until you are satisfied.

2: If pertinent, access a chakra. Is the pain or challenge related to a specific chakra? You can always work with the chakra that is located nearest the problem.

3: Allow cleansing and transformation. Request that the streams release you from issues that have settled in both the physical and subtle tissues. Allow an activation of healthy energies in the inner wheel of any chakra(s) that pertain, and then allow a complete rebalance. You can always create chakra-based affirmations or visualizations to continue and renew this healing. Close when finished.

Once you've worked on any of these subtle cardinal planes, request that the streams rebalance all planes, physical and subtle, so they can operate together.

EXERCISE 26: GAMMA GAMELINE FOR MECHANICS

If you want to beef up your mechanics while working out or during competition, go into Gamma Gameline and ask the streams to ignite that vertical flow instantly. If you are aware of a weakened mechanical area, focus there and request the entry of an extra-special boost of gamma subtle energy. That's the quick version. If you have time, ask that this gamma energy enter the three funnels of the spine and then spread throughout your physical and subtle anatomies. These are as follows:

Internal: spiritual energy. This inner channel, made of subtle energy, holds only absolute light and will instantly flood the inner wheels of all your chakras so they can assert authority.

Middle: mental energy. This middle layer, constructed from subtle energy, carries virtual light. As we covered in chapter 4, virtual light can clear emotional and mental issues, activate self-esteem and confidence, and quicken any repair needed for a mechanical issue.

Outer: physical energy—polarity Light. The outer funnel is actually your spine, but it is made of both physical and subtle energies, seen and unseen. Gamma energy can mesh these together.

As these three channels blend together, you'll find all the cardinal axes will start working together more functionally.

EXERCISE 27: QUICK SHOT OF VELOCITY

When you want to drive up your velocity, either when working on your mechanics beforehand or during game day, you only have a second, so go for it!

Conduct Sports Spirit and either psychically visualize or sense the speed or direction you need your body or a sports implement to go. Then request that an informed past-life self, an ancestral memory, or a spiritual guide respond to your need. If at some point you have already achieved the velocity you're seeking now, swiftly bring your consciousness into your first chakra and ask that the streams activate this memory-based self. Now ask that the streams unlock the powers you need and stir them all the way through your kinetic chain, from the tenth chakra up. Then go for it.

EXERCISE 28: SUBTLY SEQUENCING YOUR KINETIC CHAIN

This exercise is one you want to walk through as often as possible. It's meant to help you find physical weak spots in your kinetic chain, track them to a chakra or set of chakras, and perform clearing with the streams. If you need to uncover the exact reasons for a sticky mechanical problem, use exercise 15 to perform a deep-dive and healing.

As you'll recall, there are two ways to perceive the kinetic chain. Select the one you like and adapt it to your sport. Then move through these simple steps using either of the chains, which I've provided again here.

Sequencing Chain One
- ▸ Ankle joints (tenth chakra)
- ▸ Knee joints (tenth chakra)
- ▸ Hip joints (first chakra)
- ▸ Lumbar spine (low back; coordinates first, second, and third chakras)
- ▸ Thoracic spine (mid-back; fourth chakra)
- ▸ Cervical spine (neck; fifth chakra; upward flow reaches to sixth, seventh, eighth, ninth, and eleventh chakras)

Sequencing Chain Two
- ▸ Feet and ankles (tenth chakra)
- ▸ Knees (tenth chakra)

- ▸ Hip and pelvis (mainly first and second chakras; inclusive of third in a secondary fashion)
- ▸ Shoulders (fourth and fifth)
- ▸ Head (sixth and seventh; reaches upward and around into eighth, ninth, and eleventh chakras)

Simply conduct Sports Spirit and then immediately ask for an ongoing provision of the streams. Then walk through each of the links on the chain you are assessing. Ask guidance to do the following for each stage:

- ▸ Help you intuitively assess for strength and weaknesses in the physical segment and related chakra(s).
- ▸ Further activate the strengths through the inner wheel of the related chakra(s).
- ▸ Define, clear, and transform the weaknesses from the inner wheel of the affiliated chakra(s) to the outer wheels and then throughout the segment.
- ▸ Let you know what to work on further in the physical realm.
- ▸ Integrate and rebalance.

EXERCISE 29:
GEOMETRY FOR KINEMATIC (OR KINETIC) IMPROVEMENTS

When you are aware of a body segment that isn't working for you, take a few minutes and visualize yourself inserting the subtle energetics of a particular geometric form into that area. You can also use that form or any number of them within a corresponding chakra. If you desire, you can employ this same process with any of the kinetic chain segments or their affiliated chakras.

Conduct Sports Spirit. Affirm your own spirit, all the helping spirits—including the energy of your sport—and the Higher Spirit.

Focus on an area. Select the segment, such as a bodily area, part of your kinetic chain, a joint, or even a plane or axis that you believe needs improvement. You can also choose a corresponding chakra or a bodily area and its related chakra.

Request the correct geometric form. Ask guidance to provide you a vision of the form that would enable mechanical improvement. You might perceive it as if it is drawn on paper, two-dimensionally, or as a three-dimensional figure in your head. If you are unclear about what you would need, the following basic shapes hold these associated meanings.

> **Circles:** Any circular shape brings repair, renewal, and connection. Select a circle if your movements are disjointed, you can't connect with an aspect of your mechanical flow, or you need physical or emotional repair in regard to the segment.
>
> **Squares:** All square forms add security and strength. Use a square shape if you feel like a segment is slipping, is unable to pull its weight, has been injured or is weak, or if you don't feel like that area is empowered in comparison to others.
>
> **Triangles:** Triangular shapes unify and are also considered to be the most stable form. This means that will create steadiness. They will link the focused chakra or segment to the rest in the chain or help the other areas compensate for the part that isn't working well.
>
> **Spirals:** Spirals bring energy in or out. A clockwise spiral will add energy to the noted area. A counterclockwise spiral will release energy. If an area is weak or unable to hold its own, add energy. If it is overactive, release energy. We use spirals to create balance in a chain.

Insert with the streams. Request that the correct type and intensity of the streams insert the required form(s) into the appropriate places, and then allow integration.

Close. When you feel finished, release from this process.

Mechanics are crucial to success, but you don't have to do them perfectly. If you blend classical physics with quantum physics, subtle energy techniques can assist you with everything from increasing your velocity to stabilizing the planes and axes so critical to sports performance.

Now that you're aware of some of your mechanical needs, you can establish a great preparation program, the subject of the next chapter.

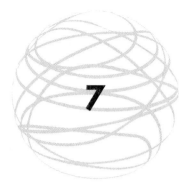

7

Athletic Preparation

The separation is in the preparation.
—Russell Wilson, NFL quarterback

Want to separate yourself from the pack in your sport and take your game to a whole new level? We've all heard the quote from Thomas Edison that genius is 1 percent inspiration and 99 percent perspiration. And it's really true—except that Thomas Edison didn't actually say those words. And what he did say referenced a different percentage.

The phrase we're all thinking of was actually uttered by an academic of the early 1890s named Kate Sanborn. By the way, she didn't provide a ratio either; she simply stated that genius is a combination of perspiration and inspiration. But talent? Talent, said Sanborn, is perspiration.[33]

Why am I going on about this? I want to make the point that no matter how much athletic talent you have—or the athlete in your life has—it's simply a starting point. The majority of your success lies in preparation, which takes perspiration.

Now I'm going to make a classist comment.

The majority of your success, however you define it, *especially* lies in preparation if you weren't born with a silver spoon in your mouth.

---

33   Ziegler, "Famous Quotes You Definitely Didn't Know Were from Women."

We'd presume, after all, that as a woman in the nineteenth century, Kate Sanborn had a steeper climb to success than Thomas Edison did. Born in the mind-1800s, Edison had an advantage in simply being a man.

I know. These days you walk a fine line when discussing issues like socioeconomic class, race, gender, sexual-gender identity, and more. I know that in times past, it was easier for White males in sports to make it than non-White males, and far easier for men over women any day. That's been changing, but there is still a singular truth: excelling at a sport takes time and money, two of the most challenging resources for the average youth or adult to come up with, and certainly for someone who is born into a socioeconomic bracket that strains pocketbooks (money) and pocket watches (available time).

I know that I shouldn't talk. I'm a White woman with a good education. My youngest son, the baseball player, is a White male who attended a private Catholic school. However, for the majority of his serious training, he only had me and my income to rely on.

I can't tell you the costs involved in supporting my son's athletics, in both money and time, when I was already a single mom running my own business with obligations to other children and to my mother.

I made a ton of sacrifices. For one, I took on extra weekend work during his high school years, for which I had to travel. He would stay at a friend's house, and that couple and their three children became his second home. I still buy the mom a Mother's Day present. If they hadn't taken him in, I wouldn't have been able to make extra money in my "off" time.

I understand the importance of pursuing a dream, no matter the soft and hard costs. You have to go for it—right? That's true for everyday athletes, elite athletes, and anybody in between.

One night when Gabe was about sixteen, I dreamed that he was playing professional ball. Actually, it appeared that he was in the majors! I decided not to say anything to him about my dream then because he had such a long way to go before that goal would be in sight.

About a week later, he told me that he wanted nothing more than to become a major league baseball pitcher.

Overwhelmed by the thought of the work involved to get him within striking distance of his goal, and knowing nothing much about baseball (as a mom in the bleachers, I gossiped through most of the games), I freaked out.

That weekend I was teaching a class in Chicago. I was talking about predictive dreams and shared my vision of Gabe. During the break, a young man came up to talk with me.

Apparently, he was a baseball pitcher. Brandon Thielk. I'm grateful to him to this day, for he said he would take on Gabe's training. He also volunteered Ryan Morris, a former Cleveland Indians pitcher. Over the next two years, Brandon and Ryan worked extensively with Gabe to align his body to support his dream. Together, they helped Gabe set a foundation he could continually build from. Without them, Gabe never would have advanced.

It still was anything but easy to pursue Gabe's (and my) dream. And if it was hard on me and Gabe, think about the challenges for kids with little parental support, money, and the like—with less opportunity.

So what can level the proverbial playing field when it comes to opportunity?

Preparation. Good old solid down-to-earth preparation.

In this chapter I'll talk perspectives and activities related to preparation, emphasizing the subtle side of preparing for sports success. We'll look at these categories: your team, your workouts, nutrition and hydration, and sleep. I'll provide lots of insights, tips, and techniques, many of which will draw upon the exercises you learned in chapter 4. I also encourage you to look back to the concepts about mechanics in chapter 6 and to create your preparation programs based on what you'll need in that regard, especially for your workouts. I'll also include vibrational remedies wherever they fit. I'll keep the advice as real and as inexpensive as possible so athletes and coaches, no matter their life circumstances, can bolster their talent without breaking the bank.

Before you design a preparation approach, however, you have to have a sense of where you want to go. The purpose of this first exercise is to create the optimum goal for your preparation. I'll refer back to it during several other exercises in this book.

EXERCISE 30: GAME DAY—
THE SUCCESS POINT OF YOUR PREPARATION

Here you will be using all aspects of your intuition to perform a visualization. The purpose of this process is to experience an optimum game day in the future.

That's right: I want you to embrace where you are headed—that over-the-top, excellent moment in which it all comes together on your mound/field/mountaintop/studio/gym/whatever. I recognize that there isn't a singular moment during which this occurs, but for the purposes of this exercise, you'll be creating one. In fact, I'm not only going to bring you to that stellar event but help you look backward in time too.

Why go to the future and use hindsight to return to "now"? To discover your best-case preparation activities. Every so often in this chapter, I'll return you to your fantastic future game day because you want to plan for the best.

As usual, conduct Sports Spirit. Ask guidance to activate all of your intuitive powers. Then sense yourself being attuned kinesthetically, verbally, and visually. The streams now lift your soul out of the here and now and drop it into your optimum future, your best game day ever.

You feel terrific! You're in the flow. You're as fit as a fiddle, without the worries of perfectionism. There is no paralysis. Any tendencies you had toward procrastination have long since disappeared.

You planned, practiced, and polished. And here you are.

Experience your success through every sense, physical and subtle. Feel the pulsing power in your physical self and how balanced and fine-tuned your emotions are. Your mind is crystal clear and focused. Your soul and spirit are in perfect alignment. You are calm and yet highly conscious.

You can hear, both intuitively and through your physical ears, what is happening for you—how your support team is cheering you on, audibly or telepathically. You can see, through your everyday and intuitive eyes, how everything has lined up—how even the natural and supernatural forces associated with your eleventh chakra are boosting you.

Sure, there are negative frequencies moving about within and outside you, but it doesn't matter. You are balanced in positivity.

From this vantage point, guidance directs your inner sight backward in time. As you peer backward through the veils of the days that led to this success point, you arrive at the exact time and space in which you started this exercise. You don't need to know all the details of what took place between that moment and your envisioned game day yet. But you now have access to every step you took—and will take—toward your achievement.

Again, acknowledge your own spirit, the helping spirits, and the spirit of your sport. Then, with gratitude, turn the remainder of your memories and abilities over to the Higher Spirit, which will begin to fill in the details of your optimal athletic preparation as you move through this chapter.

Your Team

No athlete becomes established without a team. In fact, you wouldn't be reading this book if you didn't have a team—and consider me to be a small part of it.

There are—and will be—team members who will be full-on partners, as in alive, physical, 3D, and available to you. Other participants will be far less noticeable, including your invisible spiritual guides. Maybe there's even a pet or two thrown in there! Who doesn't want a team mascot that tells you you're great no matter how your workout or diet went that day?

There will also be team associates you'll never meet, though they are very much alive. These will include the famous greats you follow on Instagram or coaches whose programs you buy and execute. Maybe you won't even be aware of certain teammates. For example, who was the mysterious person who underwrote your participation in a sports event? I once sponsored a young man for a private coach; he has no idea who provided that scholarship. Then there are the attendees in the bleachers who want to see you succeed, and you'll have no idea that it was their positive frequencies that helped get you through.

The next exercise will help you create a snapshot of the team you need right now. I recommend that you go through this process at least once a year or whenever you're ready to make another leap forward in your sport.

EXERCISE 31:
BUILDING YOUR TANGIBLE AND INTANGIBLE TEAMS

Conduct Sports Spirit and then return to your place in the future from exercise 30. Look backward through time and respond to the following questions as if you are being provided with historical information. Let your intuition fill you in. Stop as often as you need to so you can mull over a question, make some phone calls, or perform other types of research.

My Physical Team

While in a meditative state, list which of the following types of individuals in your current life are imperative to your eventual success. Also record their assignments. For instance, you might assign the jobs of tracking your gear, games, financing, or travel to a parent. Under bodily caregivers, you can list the different providers and their tasks: for example, a chiropractor for adjustments and a massage therapist for stress relief and recovery.

Team Members/Group	Assignment(s)

Coaches

Bodily caregivers

Parents or other relatives

Other authority figures

Other athletes

Friends

Indirect teachers (such as through internet programs)

Mentors I know

Mentors I don't know, such as sports figures I relate to

Others

Now review the list you just created. This time, after conducting Sports Spirit, evaluate your team members for their positivity. You want to keep interacting with those who boost your own positivity or at least neutralize your negativity. You may need to adjust the relationship to achieve this. Or, if necessary, you may want to seek out a new relationship entirely. You can evaluate who fits into which of these categories in any number of ways:

- ▸ Use your visualization tool or request insight from a guide.

- ▸ Use exercise 11, 12, or 13 in chapter 4, which employ applied kinesiology, with or without a partner. Evaluate your body's upward or downward flow in response to the name of a team member or possible team member.

- ▸ If a negative situation arises with a team member or has already come up, you can use exercise 16, Emotional Freedom Technique, or exercise 15, Energy Analysis and Healing, to clear your part of the negative relationship and then test its suitability again with applied kinesiology.

Next, create a list of the types of physical team members or groups that would be beneficial to obtain. Remember to peer backward from an optimum future. After developing this list, write a plan for how you will find these associates. Once you think that you have discovered a good contact or team member, vet them. Conduct Sports Spirit and enter a meditative state. Attune the positive frequencies inside you, then think about that figure. Do they enhance the positive energies inside or make you feel more negative? You can also double-check your findings by using applied kinesiology.

My Psychological Team

Members or groupings of this team might already be on your physical team list. That's great! You might have or need additional members, though, devoted to prepping your psychological development.

There are two activities involved in this step. The first is a pencil-and-paper evaluation of your current team and a list of still-needed team members. The second is designed to clarify the single belief that was or is in the way of your eventual and exciting achievement—the belief that is, even now, stopping you from full-on prep. Then you'll clear that belief using tools you already learned in chapter 4.

EXERCISE 32: ASSESSING OR ADDING TO YOUR PSYCHOLOGICAL PREP TEAM

Let's start putting together your mental health team.

While in a meditative state, employ Sports Spirit. Return to the listing you created for "My Physical Team." Now add any others who are currently a part of your emotional support group. Evaluate their positivity using any version of applied kinesiology (exercises 11, 12, and 13), visualization, or through a connection with guidance. As you did when developing your physical team, clear your issues with practices such as exercise 16 or exercise 15, then double-test with your own intuition or applied kinesiology.

Now jump into the future. There you are, at your success point! Ask that guidance let you know if you added particular mental health supporters as you moved through time. If so, who? What types of individuals? What roles did they fulfill? Were there any particular self-help books or processes that were essential to your success? Write down whichever ones are most applicable to this moment.

EXERCISE 33: CLEAR THOSE PREP-PSYCH ISSUES

Let's clean out that major psychological issue right now, the one that really gets in the way of your preparation activities (from the point of view of the future).

Take a few deep breaths and settle into a meditative state. For a few moments, conduct Sports Spirit. Then relate to your future happy self. Request to intuitively sense the most significant negative belief that prevented full-throttle preparation and, therefore, performance. Customize exercise 15 to this undertaking. When you are clear, request that the streams clear the issue and then ask guidance for whatever else you "did" to continue to transform that negativity.

Your Spiritual Team

In 1937 a groundbreaking book came out that included a very cool practice. The book? *Think and Grow Rich* by Napoleon Hill, a classic about making money. The exercise from it that we're going to modify involves setting up a board of directors—in this case, an invisible one.

That's right: if you desire to, you can take the role of your spiritual guides seriously by appointing them to a board of directors whose job is to provide advice. Their input will relate to your preparation activities but can also apply to other sports concerns.

How do you do this? I'll walk you through a short exercise.

EXERCISE 34: HIRE AN INVISIBLE BOARD OF DIRECTORS—YOUR SPIRITUAL TEAM

While sitting in a quiet place, grab paper and pen and conduct Sports Spirit. Activate your intuition and align with your Higher Spirit. Then request that the Spirit reveal to you at least one of the guides that is already attending you, as well as any others that can assist you in achieving your ultimate sports destiny.

You might want to imagine that you are actually sitting at a boardroom table or perhaps in an environment related to your sport. Fix this place in your mind's eye so that every time you hold a meeting, this is where your invisible team gathers.

For this first time through the exercise, write down descriptions of the board members. What are their specialties? Do they want the board to be called by a name? Also ruminate further: Are there members you'd like to invite? Request that they be issued an energetic invitation and see if they show up. Know that no matter who shows up for your spiritual team, the ultimate decisions about who its members are is up to you.

Decide how often you'd like to meet with your board and how.

The Workout: The Super Necessary Preparation

I worked with one young client who was extra keen on using subtle energy techniques. Her reason?

"I can skip my workouts and just imagine myself doing them!"

Well…life doesn't work like that. One side of the two-sided energy coin is physical, and although there are subtle perspectives and techniques you can use to hone your bodily athleticism, you'll still have to put in real time—time spent moving.

But subtle energetics can certainly make your workout routine more efficient and enjoyable, while getting you to actually do it.

A *workout* is a practice or set of exercises that enhances your athletic ability or performance. I probably didn't need to tell you that; I probably also don't have to insist that you work out. What I can emphasize is that if there is any athletic arena most apt to trigger our three failure p's—procrastination, perfectionism, and paralysis—it's this stage.

Who wants to get sweaty and feel achy every day?

Who has enough energy to totally focus on a mechanical technique while exercising? Or keep up with the nutritional diary, owning absolutely every extra slice of pizza or chocolate cake?

Who else would understand why you sometimes just freeze at the thought of going at it one more time, with that deep wonderment *Is this even helping?* that poses an athletic dilemma? After all, no matter how hard you prepare, there are no guarantees that any of that preparation will matter in the clutch of performance.

But in the end, how you're going to do on game day is all about preparation, the type that takes planning, practice, and polish.

To help you create workouts customized to your objectives, and to keep them up, I'm going to walk you through a practical exercise. Basically, it will help you evaluate a current workout and make changes, if needed, or create a new one if that's best. I'll then provide several tips related to the exercises in chapter 4 as well as vibrational remedies to get you through the grind.

EXERCISE 35: ESTABLISH YOUR WORKOUT PROGRAM

There are several stages involved in formulating a workout program. Some are practical; all make use of your intuition.

Stage One: Set Goals

After walking through Sports Spirit, ask to attune to the future self you connected with at the beginning of this chapter. Then write down at least three sets of goals you need your workouts to accomplish in these areas:

Physical. Your objective is to ensure proper form and mechanics, strength and agility, competitive musculature, and any other bodily characteristics that are vital to your sport. Review the topics covered in our last chapter to make sure you work the kinetic and kinematic chains, so you're up on your sequencing. Also evaluate how you're to keep improving the three physical cardinal planes and axes. A few tips:

> ▸ That transverse plane? Spinal rotation or limb rotation (to the sides), bench press, push-ups, chest and back flys, seated hip adduction. Go play golf!

> ▸ The frontal plane? Lateral arm and leg raises, side shuffle and side lunges, side-to-side spine bending. Take up tennis!

> ▸ The sagittal plane? Back squat, biceps curl, calf raises, front lunges, walking, and running. [34]

Psychological. Though workout programs are primarily physical, they must also cultivate mental and emotional attributes. For instance, if you'll need to hyper-focus during game day, your workout must help you practice that function of focusing. You'll learn mental and emotional tips in chapter 9 to assist you in optimizing your game day, and additional mental and emotional tips in chapter 10.

---

34   Payne, "Sagittal, Frontal, and Transverse Plane," and Sirani, "Four Easy Steps."

Spiritual. This set of workout objectives takes into account the need to fuel your soul and spirit. Meditate on the reasons you love this sport—how it fulfills you. You'll want to capture the essence of that drive in your workouts.

Stage Two: Research

After conducting Sports Spirit, undertake your research with your goals in mind. Then employ both logical and intuitive faculties, along with your real-life and spiritual connections, to create a workout program. This step also works if you already have a workout and simply need to update it. Give yourself a due date and consider analyzing the following types of data sources:

- ▸ Your own experience
- ▸ Your team—including physical, psychological, and spiritual teams
- ▸ Internet or book-based sources
- ▸ Contacts or connections
- ▸ Programs designed for others in your sport with your particular goals

Stage Three: Create a Calendar

Nothing will really happen unless future activities make it onto a calendar. Enter what you're going to do and when. As part of this step, sign up for coaching, classes, groups, and the like. Consider your circadian rhythms during this step so you can work with and not against your natural flow.

WORKOUT TIP 1: CHAIN-LOCK PREP SUCCESS

Once in a while, you get something absolutely right. And now you know that movement, thought, attitude, feeling, or approach can show up when it counts. So, chain-lock it in!

Use exercise 9, Chain-Lock. As soon you get the behavior or attitude exact, conduct Sports Spirit. Home in on these accomplishments while tapping your chest, or imagine you are tapping it. The streams will land in the inner wheel of your heart chakra. Tap a second time, and you are good to go. Now when you need that success to return, you only have to tap once again, either mentally or with a finger.

WORKOUT TIP 2: PRACTICE GAMMA GAMELINE

At least once during each workout, practice exercise 14, Go Gamma Gameline, found in chapter 4. This is especially important if the activity you're doing affects your mechanics. While focusing, also conduct Sports Spirit and ask for streams to wash into your body through the subluminal and supraluminal states, clearing any repressed or difficult emotions or beliefs.

WORKOUT TIP 3: SEIZE AUTHORITY

Okay, it's official—just admit it. You really don't want to work out.

This tip is an important one to practice because you (or the athlete you're coaching) must exercise discipline at every stage of athletics.

Conduct Sports Spirit. After taking the last step, which involves affirming the Higher Spirit, return to the sense of your own spirit. This is your higher authority, the self that knows exactly what you should be doing, when, and why.

Let your spirit infuse itself with the unlimited power of the streams, specifically requesting that they be drawn upward from the center or belly of the earth. In the middle of our planet is an amount of energy equivalent to a white star. Allow this energy to rise into your body through the inner wheel of the tenth chakra underneath the feet and be immediately shared through the inner wheels of all chakras. Now tapping into this core power of the earth, you have the energies you require to proceed.

WORKOUT TIP 4: GO WITH PROGRAMMING

Remember our discussion about programming in chapter 4? Well, you can employ that activity to get you through the toughest of workout days.

First, program the water or other form of hydration that you will consume during your workout. Conduct Sports Spirit and use your sending hand, which you determined in exercise 17, to send the streams into the fluids. Compose a statement to support your desires such as "I will adjust my speed so it matches my optimum game day" or "I'm lifting an extra pound."

Go a step further for every practice. Is there an amulet or stone that speaks to you? You might want to employ a spiritual or religious icon as a support piece, or a particular crystal to sustain an achievement. Some specifics: amethyst deflects negativity and enlivens your vision for the future; garnet or ruby bolsters your first chakra, enhancing your physical strength; and obsidian will ground you while chasing away dark thoughts. Use the same technique you would for your thirst quenchers to insert supportive statements into the stone, then keep that stone in your pocket or with your gym equipment. Clean the stone once a week or so by putting it in the moonlight overnight or sending sound through it via a singing bowl or other instrument. The cleansing will free the stone of any negativity it has absorbed. Afterward you can reprogram it for a different intention if you want to.

Want a tip for Bach Flower Remedies? Simply use them as directed. Try Rescue Remedy if you've pushed too hard or Oak if you just don't have what it takes but have to work out anyway—here comes that extra oomph! At the end of your endurance? Try Sweet Chestnut.

How about an essential oil? Mix a selected oil with a neutral carrier like almond oil and apply a few drops topically or use in an aromatherapy machine. Peppermint is great for pre- and post-workouts, and eucalyptus can be anti-inflammatory. Trying to get through the big push? A little lemon will provide extra zip.

Nutrition, Hydration, and Preparation

You become what you eat. We've all heard that phrase. Think of what that might mean if not only physical but subtle energies are part of the equation.

In this section I'm going to give you some very interesting nutrition advice. Of course, I'll cover the basics about macro- and micronutrients and hydration, every athlete's necessary considerations. You'll want to construct a nutritional plan taking your own body and sport into account. Be aware of your body type, workout regimen, caloric usage, and food sensitivities and allergies. You'll probably need to conduct your own research. The good news is that there is a lot of data in books, on internet sites, and in free apps. You can also follow the links I provide.

Then I'm going to take it to a second step. I'm going to share chakra- and subtle energy–based understandings about various foods.

You see, the differing chakras, in that they are linked with endocrine glands, can be supported with different foods. Let's say you need to really drive your first chakra. Why not assist the process with a bit of first chakra food, like a great protein? As well, various macro- and micronutrients each represent a specific type of energy. *Macronutrients* are those you need in the largest amounts. *Micronutrients* are also necessary for your well-being but are consumed in smaller quantities. I'll show you how to apply the subtle energetics of many types of nutrients, as well as fluids, as part of your technique kit bag.

Physical Nutrition: Macronutrient Requirements

There are three main categories of macronutrients. Your nutritional program ought to create the correct balance for you among these three.

> **Carbohydrates.** Carbs are broken down in the body to supply you with glucose (or sugar) to compose cellular energy. They are necessary to fuel your workouts, support your central nervous system, and make just about everything happen in your body. Usually, it's suggested an athlete get about 60 percent of their diet as carbs, emphasizing whole grains, fruits, vegetables, and beans and legumes, but you have to customize the amount to your body and your needs. I suggest you create your own standard for all macronutrients using sites including the USADA's free suggestions. This organization assists with anti-doping efforts but also with constructing nutritional plans.[35]

> **Proteins.** Proteins are vital for healthy muscles, tissues, and organs. They also boost your enzymes. They are made up of amino acids, and what's interesting is that when you eat a protein, your digestive tract breaks it into its constituent amino acids. In turn, these building blocks formulate tissue and serve as fuel. There are twenty amino acids, and foods that contain all of them are called "complete proteins." Animal proteins are complete, and so are quinoa, buckwheat, hempseed, soybeans, and blue-green algae. You can also combine foods, like whole grains with peanut butter, to create a complete protein package.

> One guideline for an athlete is to consume about 12–15 percent of their calories from proteins a day, but you really need to adjust this percentage based on your body weight.[36] Again, you can always use the USADA to obtain free insights.[37]

> **Fats.** Containing a little over twice the calories per unit as carbs and proteins, fats store energy, transport fatty-soluble vitamins, and protect your organs. There are many

---

35   USADA, "Carbohydrates."
36   Coleman, "What is the Percent of Daily Calories?"
37   USADA, "Protein's Role as a Team Player."

types of fats, and in general, you want to mainly eat unsaturated fats and limit your consumption of saturated and trans fats. Go for organic meat, fish, and dairy, oils like coconut and olive, and nuts and seeds. The typical person should get between 20 and 30 percent of their calories from fat; again, I'd recommend taking a look at the guidelines from the USADA.[38]

Physical Nutrition: Micronutrient Suggestions

There are several micronutrients, consisting mainly of vitamins and minerals, that are vital to athletic endeavors. I'm going to list the most essential for athletes and provide a few insights about their roles in the body. You can follow the links to perform free research for building your nutritional program. There are also many apps free for download that contain this material and more.

Minerals. Minerals are tiny but powerful. You need a lot of them, including.

Sodium: Maintains fluids and allows contraction of muscles.

Magnesium: Calming and aids in sleep, metabolism, and dealing with stress.

Calcium: Good for the bones and aids with testosterone and fat excretion.

Zinc: Boosts immunity, reduces inflammation, and vital for absorption.

Selenium: Prevents cell damage and aids in hormone and stress reduction.[39]

Potassium: Prevents cramping and fuels your muscles.[40]

Iron: Transports oxygen, needed for healthy muscles.[41]

Vitamins. What are the most essential vitamins for the athlete?

Vitamin B12: Energy metabolism. You'll feel weak without it.

Vitamin B6: Aids in metabolism and stress resistance.

Vitamin A: Antioxidant and for sight.[42]

Vitamin C: Decreases recovery time and keeps the immune system healthy.[43]

---

38   USADA, "Fat as Fuel."
39   Nick English, "7 Micronutrients."
40   Braun, "Potassium: Don't Sweat It!"
41   Michalcyzk, "The Best Vitamins for Athletes."
42   Ibid.
43   Peace Health, "Vitamin C for Sports & Fitness."

Vitamin K: Essential for bone and heart health.

Vitamin D: Aids with mood and bone strength, but also an essential antioxidant.[44]

My personal advice is to find a couple of supplements that can give you just about everything you need. A full-on green smoothie or healthy electrolyte or protein powder can be used to power up your micronutrients.

Physical Nutrition: Hydration

Every athlete has heard it. Hydrate! Drink water! Skip the sodas, high-octane Gatorade, and other sugary drinks and return all that water lost through the blood, sweat, and tears of sports.

In general, during and after exercise, it's recommended you drink three cups of water for every pound of water weight lost. There is a complicated formula to figure that out, which you can find at this link: https://tinyurl.com/3un9e26n. As is shared there, it's good to drink water as soon as you get up in the morning, and then drink at regular intervals before, during, and after exercising. But don't ever drink *too* much water. That can cause hyponatremia, a condition where there is a critically low amount of sodium in the blood. On the really severe end, this can cause respiratory arrest or death. You can read more about it through this link: https://tinyurl.com/mrhkbsye.

Subtle Nutrition: Macronutrient Requirements

What do the macronutrients provide on the subtle level and how can you apply this data to athletics? Let's take a look. I also encourage you to use the basic practice of programming that is provided for water in exercise 19 and do it for your food. Yes, this is why people have prayed over their food for thousands of years. You are programming the food to do good things for you!

> **Carbohydrates.** On a subtle level, carbs provide the comfort and calm you need to be grounded while preparing for or undertaking a sporty task. Yes, carbs energize, but they first create a sense of ease and that "all is well." If you overeat carbs, reflect on how your current relationship with them provides a false assurance of security and lovability. Focus on the provision of security you get when you eat a carb by requesting that the streams emphasize the serenity obtained through that macronutrient.

---

44   English, "7 Micronutrients That Are Important for Athletes."

Proteins. Proteins convey strength on the subtle level. When you just don't think you have it in you or you're scared you'll run out of your own power, go for protein. Infuse your selected proteins with power by running the streams through them. Proteins also stimulate negative reactions if you believe yourself to be powerless. Ask yourself how you became convinced you are the perpetual victim and clear that issue using exercise 15 in chapter 4.

Fats. Fats are about bonding. They connect cells and tissues together in the body, cement thoughts and actions, and hold emotions that we haven't felt yet. Because so many of our frequencies are negative, as are frequencies available outside our body, we want to cleanse the fats we imbibe so they only promote positive frequencies and outcomes. Ask for the streams to run through any fats you're eating and promote a sense of being bonded with people and energies that support you. In particular, fats can hold shame, so use exercise 16 to clear shame-based issues.

Let's say you'd like to feel unconditionally supported in your sport, such as by a spiritual guide or the Higher Spirit. That would be a good time to consume a fatty meal or snack. Before you eat the fat, ask that the streams transfer positive messages into that foodstuff. You can focus on a particular message, such as "I am only bonded to supportive people" or "I am releasing negative emotions from my body and activating healthy ones" or "I am unified with my future and successful self." You can also just let the streams carry out their influence of grace and know that you'll undo whatever negative condition lies in the system and invoke positive ideas.

Subtle Nutrition: Micronutrient Suggestions

There are a lot of micronutrients to keep track of! It can be helpful to know what each provides for your system in terms of its subtle energies. There are many ways you can work with this information.

One is to employ the streams to emphasize the subtle energies of the micronutrients you are consuming. For instance, you can use the sending hand you figured out in exercise 17 to request a specific boost for a certain supplement or food. Need strong bones? Hold your hands over a bone and send in streams while thinking something like this: "May the calcium super-strengthen my bones."

You can use your sending hand to activate all the micronutrients in, say, a blended shake. Perhaps you hold your green drink, call on the streams, think of your future successful self, and internally state, "May all these properties work for my optimum success." You don't even have to use a hand! Simply conduct Sports Spirit and ask for the streams to work for you; either that or request that your guidance do this for you.

The other option for using the knowledge about the subtle properties of micronutrients is to select those you might be missing based on their strengths. Do you feel weak when working out? Maybe you need to boost the potassium you are taking by using the streams.

Following is a list of the subtle properties affiliated with the sports-minded micronutrients.

Minerals

Sodium: Fluid performance and full-body participation in movements.

Magnesium: Achievement of flow in all aspects of life; resistance to others' negative energies.

Calcium: Strong foundation in all areas of sports; keeps mechanics stable and provides stability in general. Holds goals. Think bones. Calcium keeps your bones and attitude sound and powerful.

Zinc: Allows only positive subtle energies to reign inside you.

Selenium: Protects against internal and external negativity; releases negative thoughts into the atmosphere.

Potassium: Keeps you moving toward objectives and brings energy from nature into your muscles.

Iron: Brings subtle life energy, the stuff produced in the first chakra, throughout the body.

Vitamins

Vitamin B12: Brings natural energy throughout the body to meet your heart's desires. If you give away your energy to others, you might not metabolize this vitamin very well, so work on that pattern and keep your own vital life energy for yourself. All the B vitamins support endurance and success.

Vitamin B6: Like vitamin B12, this vitamin cycles natural energy through your system. If you tend to take on others' negative energies, however, it might not metabolize well, so clear that tendency.

Vitamin A: Maintains clear vision for your future and gets rid of whatever is in the way. Also enhances honesty in your inner sight. Can you see your strengths and weaknesses clearly? Doing so allows you to work on yourself on all levels.

Vitamin C: Keeps all levels of your physical and subtle body in flow. Also allows intimacy between you and members of your team.

Vitamin K: I believe this vitamin links you to the positive frequencies in the environment around you. It also allows you to accept and harness your personal strengths and control negative thoughts and behaviors.

Vitamin D: Literally allows your system to employ your spiritual light, the light of the spirits helping you, and the Higher Spirit's light. If your vitamin D isn't working well, you might be impacted by attachments or others' negative energies.

Subtle Nutrition: Hydration

The molecules in this nutrient carrier and cleansing agent are shaped by beliefs. Are you willing to accept yourself as pure, innocent, and loved? Let healing streams replace all lies with truths, and remember to program your fluids!

Chakra-Based Foods and Their Spiritual Messages

Following is a list of the chakras and the foods (or foodstuffs with certain qualities) that will fuel them, along with the spiritual message the chakra-related foods can deliver to you. I recommend that you experiment to see what happens if you select a chakra-specific food to eat when you're facing a chakra-specific issue. Dealing with a challenging emotion? Try a second chakra food. Program the food with the spiritual message associated with that chakra.

Chakra	Sample Foods	Spiritual Message
First	Beef, legumes, quinoa, and lean proteins and healthy fats; tomatoes, beets, radishes, cherries, and all other red or purple berries or fruits; dairy of all sorts; eggs	I deserve to be physically successful at all aspects of my sport
Second	Chicken, turkey, tofu, tempeh, almonds, salmon and other seafood; yams, sweet potatoes; whole grains; oranges, papayas, and other orange fruits	All my feelings allow me to creatively meet my athletic goals

Chakra	Sample Foods	Spiritual Message
Third	Nuts, fowl, yogurt; corn- and brown rice–based products and the squashes; also bran, barley, and sourdough bread; pineapple, bananas, and other yellow fruit; green veggies	My self-esteem and self-confidence lead to athletic achievements
Fourth	All foods related to the Mediterranean diet, such as healthy fish, lean meats, nuts; olive and avocado oils; chia, flaxseed, and whole grains; green vegetables; bright fruits	I love myself enough to accept only positive frequencies from others
Fifth	Crunchy foods and those with intense flavors; lean meats and whole grains; mineral-rich foods; blue foods such as blueberries and blackberries; spinach, seaweeds, and other mineral-based veggies	I am continually guided toward athletic success
Sixth	Fish, eggs, pork, lamb, seafoods, and nuts of all sorts; whole grains; red, brown, and basmati rice; purple foods like berries; pears and melons; organic or dark cocoa products	I can see myself succeeding
Seventh	White foods like parsnips, white asparagus, and white fish; sunshine veggies and fruits—those grown in the sun!	I am continually reaching my divine destiny in sports
Eighth	Foods that speak to your soul; choose from any of the food groups as needed	I have mystical powers that are helping me succeed
Ninth	Bee pollen, honey, foods that represent your value system, such as if you are a vegan or eat according to your cultural roots	I am in harmony with all the beings around me, which assist me in reaching my highest goals
Tenth	Make sure all foods are organic and choose those grown in or close to the ground, such as peanuts, eggplant, cucumbers, radishes, pumpkin, grains, potatoes, and watermelon	All of the earth and the environment support my athletic objective
Eleventh	Dense proteins like beef and bison, eggs or tofu, pinto or kidney beans; seeds and nuts high in minerals; any or all veggies and fruits; vibrational substances such as programmed water, tinctures, and teas	I have connections to any powers or forces needed to succeed in my sport
Twelfth	This chakra is unique to you, so this category will consist of foods that support you in all ways	I am uniquely able to become the best athlete I can be

The Soothing, Snoring Sounds of Sleep

You want to be like a successful pro athlete? Sleep. A lot.

It's said that pro athletes need between eight and ten hours of sleep a night. After all, prep is hard work. If you can fall into that nine-hour category, you'll make fewer mistakes, get fewer injuries, have faster reaction times, and have overall better performance.[45]

On a physical level, create a good sleeping environment. You need darkness and quiet; if you can't get quiet, buy yourself one of those sleeping machines that makes sleep-inducing sounds. Wind down at night with rituals, and when you can, stick to a schedule. Don't use prescription meds unless you must. Instead, investigate various types of relaxing supplements and teas.

Personally, I like magnesium L-threonate, which was discovered and patented by MIT and has been shown to slow brain aging, reduce sleep disorders, and calm anxiety. It's the only magnesium I know of that passes the blood-brain barrier to positively impact the brain. Most other magnesium transfers into the digestive tract.[46] Of course, check with a professional for your own usage, but the last athlete I recommended it to was wowed. Living on the road as he did, he said it compensated for the sleep disturbances of that lifestyle.

On the subtle level, it's important that you learn how to shift your brain waves so you can relax yourself. Brain waves are measurements of the speed of changes in the electrical charges in your brain. The faster the hertz, or cycles per second, the more active your awareness. The slower the cycle, the closer you get into sleep and then deep sleep.

One of the best tricks I teach athletes is to program their brain so they have a process for relatively quickly achieving the delta brain wave, or the deep-sleep state. But there is another brain wave under that one! It's called infra-low. Delta waves operate between .5 and 4 cycles per second, but infra-low operate under .5 cycles per second. It's in this cycling that we store our traumatic memories. Why not use your sleep time not just to rest and restore but to also work through your psychological issues, such as those that are preventing your success? Even to work through the daily stressors involved in grinding out your athletic ability? To accomplish this, you can use the next exercise, a guided meditation, to walk yourself down from a higher state of awareness into the seas of sleep, even while allowing the streams to clear your stressors in infra-low cycling.

45   Skidmore, "8 Ways to Sleep Like a Pro Athlete."
46   Life Extension, "Magnesium L-Threonate."

EXERCISE 36: CYCLING INTO A HEALING SLUMBER

About one-half hour before you're ready to go to sleep, walk through this exercise. It will program you for the deep sleep of the delta brain wave. You must move through the delta brain waves in the four phases of sleep several times a night to wake up rested and rejuvenated. This exercise will also invite the healing process of entering infra-low at some time during the night.

The intention is to practice this exercise a few times while using the chain-lock process from exercise 9 for the purpose of programming your sleep behavior. After that, you will simply need to tap your chest a few times to let your body begin relaxing until you can fall asleep. As this is the goal, there are two parts to this exercise. The first is to practice the sleep chain-lock process. The second can take over once you've employed it a few times and you just want to chain-lock yourself to slumber.

Part 1: Practice Slipping to Sleep

Prepare for bed. You've accomplished your goals and readied your bedroom. Perhaps you have a book to read. If you use sleeping supplements or teas, take them now. This exercise will program you to fall asleep in about a half hour.

Conduct Sports Spirit. Affirm your spirit, the helping spirits, and the Higher Spirit.

Accept your current state. You might be feeling calm or overexcited. Either way, that's okay. Simply be where you are, without a need to label the feelings.

Tap into the theta brain wave. The initial part of this exercise is to guide you into the theta brain wave. This brain wave cycles right above delta and is a healing state unto itself, as it enables you to be fully grounded and yet connected to your personal spirit.

As you link with guidance, ask that your body be brought into the theta brain wave, which cycles between 4 and 8 times per second. Simply tap your chest once to chain-lock the beginning of this theta-achieving process, and let yourself observe the serenity that begins to enfold. In your mind say *I am initiating theta with this tap*. I also invite you to shorten that statement after you've practiced this exercise a few times by internally declaring *Theta initiated*.

If you want to, you can tighten the bones in your head and then release them, and then do the same for every other body part all the way down to your toes.

Simply observe any thoughts you have without judgment, and if you are visual, picture yourself somewhere in nature, in a place of peace and restoration. After a few minutes, you will begin to feel slightly dizzy and perhaps a bit spacey. That is the sign that you are in theta and that the subtle energies of the earth and the heavens are balancing you. Chain-lock this state so it will be easy to assume again, and label it in your mind in this way: *I have achieved theta with this tap*. You could even shorten that statement to be *Theta accomplished*.

Program delta and the infra-low. Now tap your chest to chain-lock the initiating of delta and infra-low. Use a phrase like "Delta and infra-low initiated." You will not be formulating a second tap, as you did for theta, because this process will simply bring you into delta and then, at some point during the night when you are ready, the infra-low frequencies. Simply tap to start the process.

Some people like to read, hum, play music, or perform some other maneuver to slip into delta. Do what works for you and let go.

Part 2: Quick Process for Sleep

Once you've practiced the full-on sleep exercise just shared, you can shorten the process.

Prepare for bed and conduct Sports Spirit. About a half hour before you want to fall asleep, tap on your chest while thinking *Theta initiated*. Once you've reached that state, tap again and think *Theta achieved*.

Undertake whatever relaxing activities you like, and when you are fully ready to sleep, tap while thinking *Delta and infra-low initiated*. If you wake up at some point during the night and can't slip back to sleep, repeat the tap for initiating theta and then another for recognizing that theta has been achieved. Then tap again to initiate delta.

Preparation is where it's at. All categories are important, including assembling a team, creating the correct workout, and paying attention to your food, hydration, and sleep. In this chapter you learned ways to attend to both the physical and subtle sides of these matters.

Now that you're prepared to perform your best, it's time to learn how to help prevent and deal with a very real part of being an athlete: injury. That's the subject of the next chapter.

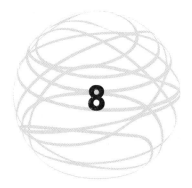

8

Injury Prevention and Care— and Speedy Recovery

Due to another back issue that required surgery, he was rarely seen on the field. (Later) In 2008... he passed Roger Clemens for second place on the all-time strikeout list...

—about Randy Johnson, former baseball pitcher

It's going to happen. It does to every athlete: injury. It could be just an annoying pulled muscle. Then there are the terrible injuries that can potentially end your playing. I've worked with clients in both categories, and every other one too.

Sometimes we don't see it coming.

About a year into the COVID-19 pandemic, Gabe contracted the disease. After he cycled through the main symptoms, including headaches, chills, fever, and a cough, the virus settled into his back. He was so stiff he could hardly move. He pushed through it, but to compensate he altered his mechanics.

For the first three months of that year, well into the beginning of the season, his pitching was all screwed up. His velocity tanked. His slider went down the drain, followed swiftly by his changeup and fast ball. Finally, Shawn Kitzman, whom I mentioned in chapter 6, drove into his college town to coach him during a series of Monday nights. Before he could get Gabe operational again, he addressed the injuries with bodywork (and so did I—long distance). Still, it took three months to get his mechanics and velocity back online. He came through it all ahead, but it was an excruciating process, physically and emotionally. For several weeks it looked like his dreams were washing away.

About a year earlier, two of his teammates underwent Tommy John surgery. One of them made it back from that, but the other never did.

Injuries are real, and they will happen. If you're reading this chapter, you've probably already struggled with at least one. If you're a coach, you might have gone into coaching because an injury stopped your forward movement toward elite playing. Injuries impact all types of athletes across the board, however. In fact, when I was walking the Camino in Portugal and Spain with friends a few years ago, we came upon a woman who was sitting at a brook and crying. Her knee was wrenched and she couldn't move it. We tended to her knee, fully expecting that she would call a taxi to finish her trip. She didn't, though. She kept going.

This woman was walking the Camino with a doll that had belonged to her deceased daughter. She'd promised to walk every step of the way in her daughter's honor. And she made it. I know she did because I saw her in Santiago, the end of the trail.

It takes perseverance to recover from (or move through) injuries and grace to figure out how to transform your life if injury means it has irrevocably changed. Sometimes you must make do for just long enough.

As another example of the latter comment, years ago I worked with an eighty-year-old man who had moved to America from China decades past. In his youth, Li Wei had loved ping-pong, also called table tennis. The sport of ping-pong has been around China since the early 1900s. Originally only rich people could afford to play it. His family had been quite wealthy and loved indulging in the local ping-pong house.

Every good memory Li Wei held about his father was intertwined with ping-pong. Then, when he was in his early twenties, his father died, and Li Wei emigrated to America. He gave up ping-pong in order to start and run his own business, and eventually to care for his own family.

Li Wei came to see me because he had a degenerative neurological disease. He wanted to complete two life goals. The first was to stand up at his granddaughter's wedding, which would take place in two months. The second was to play ping-pong one more time with his own sons.

Li Wei accomplished both goals. He had to stand upright from a wheelchair for the wedding and use a special instrument that extended from his hand to play ping-pong from his wheelchair. Before he died a few months later, he said that he was "satisfied" and that his soul could now meet his father's soul and those of the rest of his ancestors.

I didn't help Li Wei rejuvenate his muscles. I used a few hands-on healing methods to support the strength he already had, as well as some vibrational remedies. I also suggested he work with a local chiropractor who used electrical stimulation. And I helped further activate his own spirit within his body. I believe that the combination of subtle and physical activities kept his body from sliding further, while the embrace of his spirit enabled him to meet his goals.

Wherever you are injured, you can certainly benefit from the subtle energetics provided for injury prevention and care as well as for a speedier recovery. Remember that the body is the body. You might or might not fully recover, but no matter what happens, you can transform.

The Basics of Sports Injuries

In general, sports injuries are usually labeled as acute, overuse related, or chronic. From a practical point of view, these injury types can be described in the following ways:

Acute injuries: These are usually the result of a traumatic event occurring within that week. Examples include fractures, sprains, dislocation, or even off-field wounds, such as from a car accident. They can also involve immediate recovery post-surgery.

Overuse injuries: These happen over time, such as when you use repetitive motions for a sport. Included here are problems like tennis elbow, swimmer's shoulder, jumper's knee, and tendonitis.

Chronic injuries: This category includes injuries of the kind that plague you for more than three months. I include long-term recovery and care after surgery in this category.

No matter the type of injury you or the person you're coaching has, there are three stages of rehabilitation. I devote a section to each in this chapter, with a focus on subtle fixes. The stages are:

Phase One: Injury Prevention. There are a lot of ways that athletes prevent injury; among them are using safe mechanics and good equipment. I'll share a couple of subtle exercises for this in the related section.

Phase Two: Injury Care and Recovery. There are substeps to this category, and we'll cover all three in the related section.

Phase Three: Return to the Sport. You want to rush back—but sometimes you can't! What if your playing is truly altered or slow to return? How can you give yourself grace in this situation? Exercises will assist.

Phase One: Injury Prevention

The best way to deal with an injury is to never get one.

I know that's difficult. But there are a few essential subtle energy processes that can assist in this endeavor. The first is to establish and maintain strong energetic boundaries. The second is to increase body awareness. While you won't be completely immune to the challenges of your sport, with these two enhancements on your side, you'll be better able to fend off possible disasters and mitigate those that occur.

Establishing Solid Energetic Boundaries

Energetic boundaries are the sum total of the biological and subtle energy fields emanating from the various parts of the self—body, mind, and soul. Another word for this emanating field is the biofield.

The word *biofield* was assigned by a group of scientists in 1994 to describe the field of energy and information that surrounds and interpenetrates the human body. It operates in various ways, including electromagnetically and thermally, as well as through quantum fields.[47] That means this type of field fits exactly into our theme of the book: it is both physical and subtle.

We each have a unique bodily blueprint, made of sound and light, and the same goes for our biofield.[48] If our biofield pulses to the song of our soul, we will be attuned to the environment. We'll naturally operate from our internally positive frequencies and relate to the externally positive ones. When this field is weaker, such as if we're tired or feeling down and out, our energy field will be more vulnerable to others' negativity. We can lose mental and physical focus, and when that happens, we make mistakes. That means we can more easily get injured all on our own, but we also become susceptible to responding to the harmful desires and moods of others.

47   Zahran, "Human Bio-field and Psychical Sensitivity."
48   Ibid.

It's been shown that our own biofield is strongest and most supportive of our natural decision-making style when we're by ourselves. In contrast, when we're around someone showing strong emotions or in a crowd exhibiting a shared response, we can get deterred. Information can transfer into us and overwhelm us. That angry tennis foe? Her potent emotions might not only make you miss your stroke but be vulnerable to her 150-miles-per-hour ball, which could ram your chest. If there are dozens or hundreds or thousands of "bleacher people" against your succeeding, it's easy to understand why it's so important to have a solid biofield.

Then there are the invisible forces that go bump in the middle of the night, like ancestral hauntings or attached entities. How about the liabilities involved with curses, energy markers, or other energetic constructs?

It's on you to create the right workout and lifestyle conditions to prevent injury. Check out your equipment. If you can't afford new, buy the best available at used sporting goods stores. No matter what, however, you'll benefit from establishing energetic boundaries. To accomplish that, I encourage you to use the following exercise a few times a month.

EXERCISE 37: PUTTING SUBTLE ENERGY CRYSTALS IN YOUR ENERGY FIELD

This technique is based on classic research on crystals grown in a laboratory.

Science shows that crystals can be programmed so that their atoms respond in certain ways: within a set time, in reaction to specific events, or both. This means that by using energy work and the streams, you can actually create subtle crystals that operate in the following ways:

Time crystals: These types of crystals create specific states of matter that repeat over a certain amount of time. Actually, the atomic patterns regenerate in a specific time period. The application of this is that you can potentially program "subtle crystals" with programs that will go off at set times. In terms of injury prevention, the idea is to set subtle energy crystals in your biofield that will trigger every so often to strengthen your field so it is less vulnerable to your own negative programs or to others' attacking energies or destructive moods.

Space crystals: These crystals are made of atomic patterns that hold or trigger during specific events. The application is that you can program a subtle crystal to go off under certain conditions—such as when a batter walks to home base or tries to barrel into you while you're holding third.

Space-time crystals: Crystals in which the atomic patterns regenerate in a certain time period and after a set event. Space-time is essentially four-dimensional, so you are attempting to create a reaction in the third dimension.[49] This means you can put energetic crystals in your field that will both keep it powerful and ward off negative intrusions.

It's easier to create these subtle crystals than you might think. Just walk through the following process.

After conducting Sports Spirit, call the streams to you. While noting their incoming power, intuitively stretch into your surrounding biofield. Be open to areas that feel strong or dynamic and others that seem weak or thin. You might sense the presence of holes, attachments, or holds, and even be aware of phantom beings or the dislike or disapproval of people who wish harm to your athleticism or well-being.

Now request that guidance form subtle crystals out of the streams. Envision these beautiful points of light and sound as they are programmed for time and space to cleanse your field on a regular basis and fend off any persons, energies, or intrusions that could cause injury. These crystals will remain in your energy field. You can renew them any time you desire. Close when ready, and feel how much stronger you are.

Increasing Your Body Awareness

The more body awareness you possess, the easier it will be for you to keep your body out of harm's way. Here's an exercise that can help.

Your soul and body are meant to be as one. As figure 1 on page 32 shows, your spirit ties these aspects of self together even as it manages your mind.

One of the byproducts in this "how it's supposed to be" scenario is that you can invite your body to be simultaneously calm and alert, the perfect state for avoiding injurious events.

---

49   Wilczek, "Crystals in Time."

There is an Eastern label for this way of being: *samadhi*. This is a profound state in which we're absorbed in the Absolute, completely rapt and joyful, but also in full awareness of our mental and physical capacities. In other words, we're both serene and "on" at the same time. Individuals in this state sometimes report that time seems to slow down, they are able to see what's going to happen, and even though time is moving quickly in the outer world, they feel like they have "forever" in which to decide how to act. In other words, samadhi equals flow, the perfect state in which to be athletic.

How can you get yourself in flow? The following exercise will help you enter that state and return to it should you lose it—which we all do. As with most important activities, such as holding an intention (which we discussed in chapter 7), you must practice—and practice and practice. Run through the previous exercise first; you'll want subtle energy crystals already placed within your field for this one.

EXERCISE 38: INJURY PREVENTION WITH BODY AWARENESS

Conduct Sports Spirit and request that the streams be provided to encourage flow. Know that through your intention, these streams will also unify the highest elements of your body, mind, and soul with your personal spirit. Now bring your consciousness as quickly as possible to your center of gravity, which you learned how to obtain in exercise 23. Ask that the streams hold you in this center of gravity or simultaneously in your central chakra and your bodily center of gravity.

Key to achieving samadhi or flow is emanating from the middle wheel of this center of gravity. It doesn't matter if you're actually based in a bodily part or a chakra; the absolute light is present everywhere. Request that guidance use this absolute light to stimulate your unique blueprint. The codes of that blueprint then spread throughout all aspects of you, including your external energy field. Those subtle crystals you placed in the last exercise now resonate with who you are across all time and space. You are now in samadhi, aware of self and other, and power is always available to you for athletic prowess.

Phase Two: Subtle Energy Injury Care and Recovery

There are actually many substeps to this category. To work on them, I'm going to provide a single overarching exercise called Psychic Surgery. Then you'll also be walked through several add-on exercises, many of which can apply to all phase two stages. I'll also include an exercise specific to each of these stages.

- ▸ **Protection and offloading.** This stage is safeguarding the wounded area to prevent additional damage. It also supports the body in resting the injured tissue, especially while inflammation increases during the first few days.

- ▸ **Safe recovery of motion and strength.** During this stage, you begin to use the injured part of the body again in a careful way. It's vital to reintegrate any injured segments into the kinetic chain during this time period.

- ▸ **Reconditioning.** Now you have to modify your usual conditioning or workout program, reexamine and fine-tune your mechanics, and use pain as a baseline for activities.

Clearing Negative Forces and Activating Positive Forces for Injuries

You've worked with forces many times before this, starting in chapter 4. No matter what type of injury yours is—acute, overuse, or chronic—or where you are in the process of injury care and recovery, you can always benefit by clearing negative forces and subtle charges and activating healing energies.

This next all-encompassing exercise might stop with the healing of the obvious injury or deepen into resolving earlier maladies. As an example of the latter possibility, I'll tell you about Jamie, a college soccer player I once worked with.

Following a concussion Jamie suffered on the field, she rested for the prescribed amount of time and then was cleared to play. But a year later, every time she was in the same position on the field where she'd been hurt, she was felled by a terrible headache. Together we discovered that she was reexperiencing an aspect of herself that was still in a shock bubble from an injury deliberately inflicted by her brother: in a fit of jealousy, he had thrown a baseball at her head, and the subtle energies of his rage were still locked into Jamie. Once we processed that primal wound, she stopped getting the headaches.

Of course, you might track an injury reaction to an even earlier time period. I once worked with a track and field star who was trying to recover from chronic knee pain. The doctors and physical therapists couldn't figure out why Chloe's knee still acted up; her tests were clear. We tracked the problem to a past life. She'd been a runner for a tribe, specifically in charge of warning about danger. She once tripped when trying to reach her tribe to warn them of an invasion and was delayed. Because she didn't arrive in time, her people were wiped out. Her shame and guilt were stuck in her knee. It took her a few months to clear out those emotions, but eventually her knee stopped giving her pain.

Technically, I call the process you're going to do "psychic surgery." I know—many of us relate this term to the healers who reach into a client's body to pull out nails, tumors, or clots of blood. The psychic surgery I'm referring to is actually simpler (and less messy) than that. It involves eliminating or reducing a subtle energy template that produces a harmful effect and adding or activating a subtle template and codes that can repair and build.

A template is a pattern that holds either negative, neutral, or helpful subtle energy codes. Think of it as a kind of mesh that impacts the areas it lies within. I find that an injury sometimes doesn't clear because there is a template made of thoughts, feelings, experiences, attitudes, and our own and others' negative subtle energies keeping it in place. To clear a challenging template and bring in and activate a new one, we'll be working with the ninth chakra. That's the golden chakra over your head that you tap into during Gamma Gameline. As you might remember, it holds all the soul codes that are best for you. Once in your subtle and physical system, these can release negative codes and formulate best-case templates.

Here is a reminder of the various core spaces and places you might need to work.

Possible Sources of Issues

Time Frames

- ▶ Ancestral
- ▶ Past life/lives
- ▶ In between lives
- ▶ Childhood
- ▶ Adulthood

- Chakra based:
  First (womb to 6 months)
  Second (6 months to 2½ years)
  Third (2½ to 4½ years)
  Fourth (4½ to 6½ years)
  Fifth (6½ to 8 years)
  Sixth (8 to 14 years)
  Seventh (14 to 21 years)
  Eighth (21 to 28 years)
  Ninth (28 to 35 years)
  Tenth (35 to 42 years)
  Eleventh (42 to 49 years)
  Twelve (49 to 56 years)

The chakras then recycle every seven years, starting with age 56, which locates in the first chakra.

Forces

- Environmental
- Physical
- Psychological
- Digital
- Spiritual
- Missing

Pathway issues

Stuck subtle charges/others' energies

Attachments (cords, curses, energy markers)

Holds (deflection shields, miasms)

Nature of the block

Assess whether it is primarily in any one or more of these sites:

- Physical/body
- Subtle: chakras, auric fields, meridians, nadis, or overall subtle

- ► Emotional

- ► Mind: lower or higher

- ► Soul

EXERCISE 39: PSYCHIC SURGERY

Now for the psychic surgery steps.

Conduct Sports Spirit. Affirm your own spirit and those of others, including the spirit of your sport, and then relate to the Higher Spirit.

Focus. What injury would you like to analyze or send healing energies to? Be clear about this.

Request the streams. Ask guidance to provide streams to activate your intuition so you can unlock all the causal issues in your injury and bring a healing template on board.

Intuit the cause. You'll remain in this stage for as long as necessary, as you might be peeling away several layers of causal issues.

Begin by focusing on the apparent cause of the wounding. When did it happen? How? What forces were involved, as well as subtle energies? Is there a self still in a shock bubble? Let guidance and the streams release this self and provide new boundaries, even as this injured self is being reintegrated. Know that the streams are clearing entrance or exit points, infused negative subtle energies, and the pathway. Now request that the streams be sent from above your ninth chakra and all the way downward into your physical and subtle bodies. Inside—and in your biofield—they will release you from negative energies and their templates. The incoming healing codes will activate or establish new patterns or templates to transform you at all levels.

If you sense that the wounding is deeper (and earlier) than the most recent event, keep requesting that guidance take you back in time, further and further. Then repeat the steps in the last paragraph until you feel fully transformed.

Ask for more streams. Request that the same or additional streams keep providing healing and insights, even as they integrate the positive energies and templates into all parts of you.

Close. Return to your life when ready.

EXERCISE 40: HANDS-ON HEALING FOR PSYCHIC SURGERY

Sometimes you can bump up the impact of your injury-healing efforts by using your hands. You learned how to do this in chapter 4 and exercise 17, so use that knowledge with these tips, each of which should be conducted after Sports Spirit.

Acute injury. As soon as you can after receiving an injury—or if you're around an athlete who is injured—turn on your sending and receiving hands. Request streams and ask that all healing properties be immediately available. Forces and subtle energies are cleared; positive templates are brought in and activated. Guides will remain present to reinforce this process.

Ongoing injury. Use the chain-lock idea, and when you sense that there is pain in the injury site or that it needs reinforcement, touch that area (or imagine touching it) with your receiving hand. Out go the reasons for the pain. Then touch it again, in real life or in your mind, focusing on your sending hand. Needed and healing energies go in.

Chronic injury. Twice a day request that streams simultaneously flow through your sending hand and into the injury area. They will bring in healing energies, which will in turn pull out harmful energies. These will be drawn to your receiving hand, although they won't actually go through it. Rather, they will stream around that hand and be released into the general world to be rehabilitated.

For all injuries. Program your water or other liquids! As you were shown to do in exercise 19, request that healing streams bring absolute light of the highest nature into your liquids in order to continue healing your injuries and strengthening the bodily areas that are absorbing new stress.

EXERCISE 41: ELEMENTAL HEALING

Fire can burn out microbes. Earth fills in tissue wounds. Stone bonds bone cells together, and so on. What am I talking about? Listed below are a handful of the ways to employ the subtle elements introduced in the "Your Essential Elements" section on page 134. I often employ subtle elements to enable quicker healing. After all, the physical and subtle bodies are formed from subtle elements, which in turn enable the existence of muscles, tissues, bones, and all parts of your system. Following are the ways I use the subtle elements. You can then walk through an exercise with which to apply these elements.

Element	Healing Qualities
Fire	Burns out microbes and decreases mast cells: immune cells made by the bone marrow that increase the histamine and cytokines causing inflammation
Water	Cleanses tissue, provides buffering around a new injury, and washes away toxic emotional or physical buildup in ongoing or chronic injuries
Air	Clears out the lymph system and invites guides to bring you instructive messages
Earth	Builds and repairs tissues; fortifies wounds so they can heal
Metal	Deflects others' negative predictions and medical statistics that are not in your favor; keeps you conscious of your power
Stone	All stones hold historical data and can be programmed to carry out specific functions, but their abilities vary by the geographic origin of the stone and its type. For instance, an amethyst geode in Africa will hold the natural history of that region; one from Brazil will act like a library for its site. All amethysts deflect negativity and carry spiritual truths. Once you own an amethyst, it might start storing data about you. In the same vein, a quartz will hold data from its original region and can store and direct spiritual energies for anyone using it.
Wood	Renews injured tissues, calms nerves
Ether	Helps you settle into a sense that it will be all right and you are to look at the bigger picture
Star	Empowers your passion for the sport
Light	All types and colors of light deliver love; love is the great healer
Sound	All types of tones of sound increase power; power keeps you moving
Presence	The energy of the Higher Spirit; allows you to be your own "I Am"

Have a sense of which of the many elements to direct toward a concern? Even if you don't, you can use this process:

After conducting Sports Spirit, focus on your injury. You can also embrace the feelings related to this injury or the after-care process. Then request that the streams pick up and transfer into you the elements needed to provide support and healing. You can request specific elements or allow guidance to choose for you. Remain in connection with the resulting sensations until you feel like disengaging, knowing that the streams will remain linked and operational.

EXERCISE 42:
USING VIRTUAL LIGHT TO QUICKEN HEALING

As we covered in chapter 4, virtual light constitutes quantum fluctuations. That grand term means that virtual light can shift possibilities into probabilities. Because of this, I often employ the streams to help the physical body repair as fast as it can.

Typically, I invite clients to engage the virtual light in the center of the chakra nearest the injury. Deep in the middle wheel is absolute light, surrounded by layers of virtual light, and then the polarity light on the outer wheel. If you don't know which chakra to employ, you can always focus inside the heart chakra and allow the virtual light to be spread throughout the system. You can also refer to the subtle elements shared in the previous exercise and invite streams to accelerate the effects of any of those elements.

For instance, like Gabe, I was infected by COVID-19. As soon as I realized I was getting ill, I immediately inserted virtual light into the streams and sent them throughout my body. Two days later, although still tired, I was feeling healthy again. I also used the same process to bring the fire element throughout to burn out the virus, and I believe that's one reason I didn't have any long-term symptoms.

The process is simple:

After walking through Sports Spirit, ask guidance to send the streams through your best-case source of virtual light to activate that energy. Then invite the streams to be directed into and around the injury site and any other important aspect of the body (physical and subtle), mind, or soul, thus encouraging quicker healing. All negative side effects will be mitigated. Also request that any of the subtle elements already present, or that should be introduced, be sped into quick action with either these streams or new streams. When you feel like your healing is in motion, acknowledge that the process will continue and return to your everyday life.

EXERCISE 43:
IMMEDIATE PROTECTION AND OFFLOADING

You can run through this exercise within days of being injured, post-surgery, or in case of re-injury.

Conduct Sports Spirit and request an immediate delivery of the streams. They will surround the injured area like a spider web, serving as a bandage by providing the boundary needed to stop further damage. The streams will also deliver all the elements needed to cushion you from pain, support the self in the shock bubble, and instantly wash away others' imploded and negative subtle energies. Simultaneously, all forces and pathways will be cleared. Streams will be provided to assist the rest of the body with adapting to the shift in balance caused by an injury and to assist in the healing process.

Phase Three: Return to the Sport

Here are some exercises for phase three to help you safely return to the action.

EXERCISE 44:
SAFE RECOVERY—MOTION AND STRENGTH

You're up and at it again. You're tentatively using the injured area and perhaps even building your strength. Reconnect that bodily segment to the rest of your kinetic chain to heighten recovery and decrease the possibility of re-injury in this way.

After walking through Sports Spirit, think about the entirety of your kinetic chain. If you need a refresher, review that knowledge in chapter 6. What part of the chain is in most need of recovery? Which chakras are linked to it? With this information in mind, request that the streams insert the elements necessary to reestablish a bond between that segment/chakra and all others. Simultaneously sense the strengthening of your biofield. You can go through these steps as often as needed.

EXERCISE 45: RECONDITIONING

You're getting back to being you! Now you want to use pain to monitor your activities but still push just enough to recover. So return to exercise 13, Applied Kinesiology to Use the Body's Flow, in chapter 4. While attuned to your body, and just before performing an activity, sense whether your body's energy moves up for a yes or goes downward for a no. Conduct a movement if you sense a yes, and don't if it's a no. Is your response neutral? Go slow and test it out. Once you've made a move that works great, chain-lock it in as you were taught in exercise 9 in chapter 4.

Post-Injury: Return to Your Sport

If you're returning to your sport in some capacity, you might expect to feel happy, but that doesn't always happen.

It's really easy to judge ourselves because we're not living the happily-ever-after. Sure, we might be thrilled that we're gaining ground again. But we might also be out of shape, out of kilter, and just plain out of sync. Some of us might never be what we once were, and we must deal with that fact. The following exercises will help you with these various possibilities.

EXERCISE 46: VISUALIZE YOUR RETURN

We covered visualization in chapter 4. It's a vital tool to retrain your body and ease your mind when you're getting back on the field—or wherever your game is played. Walk through all the steps of visualization after you conduct this one important step:

Look forward, not backward.

It would be easy to play an old tape and think you'll be what you once were. But history never repeats itself. So spend time constructing a new vision for how you will look and feel when you're fully recalibrated. That's the movie you want to play when you're visualizing. Know, too, that you can keep changing the movie as you move forward. It's your life and your future.

EXERCISE 47: GO FOR FREEDOM

You learned how to tap, or perform EFT, in chapter 4. As you reengineer your life post-injury, commit to tapping out your fears and judgments every day. Hold for the vision you created in the last exercise and keep clearing as you go. Typical fears include these:

- ▸ Re-injury

- ▸ Decreased confidence

- ▸ Being overwhelmed by the loss and grieving you've experienced

- ▸ Performance anxiety

The other thing to keep in mind is that different can be better! I worked with a client who was out of basketball for a year and then took six months to regain his full power. Guess what? By the time that year and a half were over, he had improved his performance beyond what he could do before.

EXERCISE 48: PROGRAMMING THROUGH YOUR EYES

Any time you are rebuilding after injury or just plain seeking to improve your performance, it can take months or even years to retrain in order to achieve your physical or technical goals. Typically, the body needs a lot of time to practice the new signal between the brain, muscles, and tendons to create an improved movement.

Is there a faster way?

As it turns out, there is an easy technique to simply "program" the body to move in a new way. This process is taught by Liz Larson, who works through Cognomovement Therapy, a company that provides high-level chakra knowledge to improve performance, amongst other activities.

If you know how to access the brain and the correct pattern in the muscles, Larson teaches that you can teach the body the new movements instantly and permanently. The eyes, the brain, and the spinal cord are one unit, and all nerves are accessible through this system. Want to change the pathway of the nerves? Utilize the eyes. Try it out! Follow these steps, start with your warm-up stretch, and see how it goes.

Test: Try your first warm-up stretch and measure how far you can reach. For example, touch your toes.

Assess: Carefully notice which muscles are needed to perform this move. For example, do you feel your hamstrings pulling or are the muscles in your low back also involved?

Visualize: Picture yourself performing this movement in a new and improved way. For example, you can reach your knees now, but you want to reach your feet. You are showing the body what you want it to do.

Change: While standing or sitting, normally move your eyes in an exaggerated figure 8. The idea is to stretch them as far to the left, right, top, and bottom of your eye socket as they can go. This stretch is a little uncomfortable but aids in changing the communication between your brain and body. Do this at least three times.

Test: Try the initial exercise once again and see what has shifted. Note your progress. What can you do now that you couldn't before?

Repeat: Do this process again until you have achieved the result you want. Try it again with another movement that you want to change quickly.

Stones and Oils for Any Injury

Remember talking about the various crystals and essential oils you can use for sports performance? Well, you can apply the same knowledge—and the ways to wield it—to injuries. In particular, you can inhale an oil directly or put a few drops in a bath, in a warm or cold compress, or in massage oil.

The following chart offers suggestions for acute, overuse, and chronic conditions. These ideas can be applied whether you're in injury care and recovery or returning to the sport.

Remedy	Acute	Overuse	Chronic
Stones	Amethyst: Reduces pain and speeds up healing process Moonstone: Enables grieving for the self in the shock bubble Carnelian: Alleviates trauma Pearl: Stabilizes Tiger's eye: Grounds; aids in reducing disassociation	Rose quartz: Anti-inflammatory Bloodstone: Alleviates strain Chrysocolla: Relieves muscle tension Amber: Rebalances Smoky quartz: Pulls out negativity	Hematite: Reduces stress and nerve pain Turquoise: Invites spiritual messages about how to help condition Malachite: Pulls out long-term inflammation and negative beliefs Citrine: Returns confidence Variscite: Reduces chronic pain
Oils	Peppermint: Anti-inflammatory Lavender: Calms and relaxes Arnica: Releases trauma Lemongrass: Quickly releases inflammation and swelling Eucalyptus: Clears and opens pathways	Helichrysum: Relieves spasms Marjoram: Relaxes tension Ginger: Warms muscles and lessens stiffness Clary sage: Promotes relaxation Frankincense and myrrh: Reduces joint pain	Yarrow: Returns to balance, reduces inflammation Black cumin: Reduces long-term pain Rosemary: Antioxidant, helps carry away toxins Rosehip: Manages pain Juniper berry: Relaxation

There are three main types of injury: acute, those caused by overuse, and chronic. There are also three main stages of dealing with injury: injury prevention, injury care and recovery, and the return to the sport. In this chapter, chock-full of examples, you learned several subtle energy techniques to help you address injury at all levels.

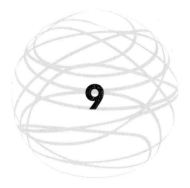

9

Game Day

Champions keep playing until they get it right.
—Billie Jean King, former tennis champion

It's your moment—or day, week, event, or goalpost. There are many different types of game days, but every sport has one.

The circumstances under which you get to pull it all together.

The presentation of the skills you've been honing.

The moment you get to show yourself—and maybe a corner of the world—what you've been accomplishing.

A game day might be a competition with others or a trek just for you. Thousands might watch you perform or maybe no one will at all. Soon I'll be hiking across France on a long-distance walk that will only be witnessed by a single friend, and yet those ten days will be an important "game day" for me. Game days can include try-outs, a final show of skill, or, if you're a coach, an event featuring your student.

As you know, each game day comes with its own unique set of challenges. You can somewhat control the lead-up—your planning and prep. But the actual moments of performance stress are fairly uncontrollable. Depending on your sport, the topsy-turvy factors might include weather, competition, bystanders, your own mood and physicality, and even the amount of sleep you got the night before. No matter what, though, you have to put on a brave face, even if you don't feel like it.

And sometimes, we really don't feel like it.

I once worked with a professional European soccer player who was scared to death about a Saturday game, mainly because he hadn't slept well for days. Why hadn't he? Because his grandmother was dying.

Energy work can help in a situation like that, and that's what this chapter aims to do. I'll start with a section about game day preparation, in which I'll emphasize subtle techniques. Then I'll offer practices to do right before and during a performance. I'll also share a bit about post-game strategies and ways to use everything from subtle elements to vibrational remedies. In the end, it's important to keep game day in perspective. No matter how that moment in time goes for you, you are bigger than any single moment.

Preparing for Game Day

You read an entire chapter about preparation. This section is different: it's about game day preparation, which is a beast unto itself.

When do you start prepping for game day? If you're like most of the athletes I've worked with, it's when you become aware of the butterflies.

In the case of a cheerleader I assisted, she started feeling nervous two days before a meet or a football game. She'd struggle to eat healthy food—got to love those carbs when you're scared, right? She wouldn't sleep well. She'd drift off in class. We had to come up with subtle processes for her to use up to three days before her game day situation as her butterflies zipped around her belly like tiny armored trucks.

On the other hand, I worked with a martial arts teacher who put on competitions for his students. He didn't sense his butterflies until an hour before an event began, but these butterflies were much more beneficial than most. As he shared, "I don't exactly get 'nervous.' It's more like some greater part of me kicks into high gear, and I become super aware of everything I'm doing."

His butterflies weren't flying in fright. They endowed him with a sense of excitement, which is the opposite side of the fear coin.

There are many ways we can work with our feelings and the time leading up to game day, and I'll present them for you. If you can, walk through these exercises in the order provided, as they build on each other.

EXERCISE 49:
TRANSFORMING YOUR FEELINGS AND AWARENESSES

Your feelings are on edge. Whether it's several days or a few minutes before your grand appearance, it's time to use subtle energies to change potentially draining feelings into supportive and creative ones. Just flow with these steps.

After completing Sports Spirit, call on the streams. Use them to locate and settle within your center of gravity. If your main chakra is in a different location from your center of gravity, link your center of gravity and your main chakra with the provided streams. Then access your intuition and focus on each of your feelings and awarenesses, one at a time. You'll be checking to see whether you're being affected by any of the feelings in the list that follows. If an unsettling feeling is present, stop for a few moments and nestle with the feeling, allowing the streams to transform it from its negative underbelly into its life-enhancing upside.

Unsettling Feeling or Awareness	Transformed Feeling or Awareness
Fear or nervousness	Excitement or thrill
Anger or resentment	Physical and mental power
Obsessiveness (such as perfectionism)	Flexibility/self-acceptance
Negativity	Stimulation to achieve
Fear of failure	Joy for the sport
Fear of success (such as fear of others' envy)	Knowledge of being "good enough"
Burnout	Ease and relaxation
Desire to be admired	Meeting of self's goals
Insecurity	Relaxed attitude
Laziness/avoidance	Excitement to show up and learn

How might this evolution of feelings really work? I once helped a college swimmer who started obsessing about every little thing a few days before a meet. Every time he caught himself ruminating, even about what suit to wear or if he'd shaved close enough, he asked for the streams to change the obsessiveness into flexibility and self-acceptance. And it worked! He began to feel looser before every competition and started to excel more often than not.

Visualization

It really works to visualize success on your game day. Use the process described in exercise 10, which also employs the chain-lock activity. Specify how many times a day—and for how many days—you want to visualize an optimum performance. If you have a particular activity that scares you, see yourself accomplishing the task successfully. It's also helpful to build in a few "oops" moments: experience yourself making a mistake or being slow on the draw, and practice patience and polishing.

Set a Board of Directors Meeting

How might you benefit from your spiritual team? Recall that you established a board of directors in exercise 34. If you haven't walked through that exercise yet, now would be a good time to do so.

Assemble the board and request that they prepare you for the upcoming game day. Is there anything else you need to plan for, practice, or polish? Have you been getting too perfectionistic or have you been feeling paralyzed? Are you procrastinating, putting off anything that must be done? Finally, request the presence of any board member who could uplift you on your actual game day.

EXERCISE 50: DEEP DREAMING

We can often work through our fears about performance during our sleep, especially when in the deep state of infra-low that we discussed in chapter 7. When preparing to sleep, run through that chapter's exercise 36, Cycling Into a Healing Slumber. Before walking through that half hour of sleep prep, write down whatever is plaguing you about your upcoming performance and request that your own inner spirit work it through while you're sleeping. Pay attention to any dreams that arrive, and work with them the next day.

In general, there are three types of dreams, and they can be processed in these ways:

Psychological. You can use psychological dreams to move through an issue. You'll awaken from these dreams with a strong sensation or feeling.

To make use of a psychological dream, consider that every part of the dream represents an aspect of you. Get out a pen and some paper and write down every element of the dream you can remember. Then go into a meditative state. Interact with each subject or element and write down what it means. What does that part of you represent? What message is it providing you? How is it helping you work through a challenge in regard to your performance? Add up all the pieces and you'll have the insight you need.

Visitation. Sometimes a guide or advisor shows up in a dream. These types of dreams won't feel psychological. You'll sense that the visitor is real and genuine and was meant to impart an important statement. Take in this information and use it.

Lucid. There are certain dreams in which we are aware of being asleep, and yet we are also conscious. These dreams are meant to assist us in working something through—in making a change for the better. If you don't feel like the interactions were resolved during the lucid dream, spend a few minutes when awake reviewing what did occur, and then finish the dream through your imagination. Create an outcome that is supportive of your upcoming game day.

EXERCISE 51: DO YOUR GROUNDING

At any point—but for sure right before you're going to perform—you must ground. You learned a lot of techniques in chapter 6 to enable this, including exercise 20, Grounding for Pulling In and Pushing Off, and 23, Stabilizing Your Center of Gravity. You can use those or perform an action that is just this simple:

After moving through Sports Spirit, ask for the streams to lock you into your center of gravity, which will also be connected to your central chakra. Then let those streams wash through the inner wheels of all of your chakras and link your entire self in a vertical shaft to the center of the earth. The middle of the earth is similar to a white dwarf star, rich and full of absolute light. The streams will carry that absolute light upward and into your body, from the tenth chakra upward, while gathering the desired subtle elements along the way. These also emanate into your energetic field, enclosing you in safety and strength.

On Game Day

Performance can be a short or a long haul. You might be a runner or bicyclist who goes the distance or a closer in baseball and get a single inning. How about the length of time involved in being a cross-country skier? A yoga instructor? No matter your sport, you will have a game day and a desire to perform.

In this section, I'm going to provide a number of exercises you can conduct on game day. Many of these are optional, although it's good to practice them before they are needed. At the least, however, I would recommend following this protocol before you are actually ready to perform.

- ▸ Get grounded. Use the exercise just shared.
- ▸ Breathe deeply, visualize success, and perform chain-lock in order to lock in your best mechanics and reactions.
- ▸ Lock into your center of gravity and link it with your central chakra, if that's in a different location from your center of gravity.
- ▸ Give yourself an affirmation.
- ▸ Use the streams to deactivate internal negative frequencies and bring in only positive frequencies from the environment.
- ▸ Enter Gamma Gameline. Remain in this state throughout the performance.

There are other exercises you can do both right before and then during your performance, which I'll share next. As we discussed in chapter 2, the vagus nerve is part of an apparatus that manages your fear, fight, flight, and fawn stress reactions. Stimulating your vagus nerve is also a secret weapon for fighting game day stress.

There are several ways to stimulate the vagus nerve in order to counteract stress. You see, when it freezes up, you stay stuck in a stress or trauma response. That means you want quick ways to loosen up that nerve, which in turn will loosen *you* up.

One of the best-known ways involves the movement of your eyes. I've adjusted several well-known vagus nerve eye exercises so that the one that follows is fast enough for athletes.

EXERCISE 52: STIMULATING YOUR VAGUS NERVE

Loosen up your vagus nerve by quickly affirming Sports Spirit. Then, equally fast, ask for the streams. They'll go where they are needed. Now stare straight ahead and then focus your eyes down and to the left for a couple of seconds. Come back to center for a couple of seconds, and then shift your eyes down and to the right. Return to center. You can conduct these eye movements a few times. If you've already entered Gamma Gameline, you're strengthening that vertical flow, and even if you haven't, you've helped yourself exit stress.

Added Tips for the Vagus Nerve

When you don't have time to move your eyes from side to side, set an intention and use one or more of these processes to quickly rebalance yourself.

Breathe slowly. Then slow your breath down even more. Using exercise 1, the Four-Six Breath, focus on moving your breath into and out of your abdomen.

Splash cold water on your face. That's right: cold water contracts the nervous system, helping you reset from stress into ease. If there is no way you can do this unobtrusively, sprinkle cold water on your wrists.

Go belly loud. If appropriate, make a loud noise from your belly. A belly laugh is great, but again, it might not fit the situation, so think lion's roar or elephant's trumpet. Can't do that either? Okay, *imagine* yourself making the sounds.

Chant. Go ahead. You can even do it inside your head! Use *Om*, the sound of the universe. It's been scientifically shown to be a sound that stimulates the vagus nerve and deactivates the limbic or stress system.[50]

---

50 Anxiety Recovery Centre Victoria, "Vagus Nerve Exercises."

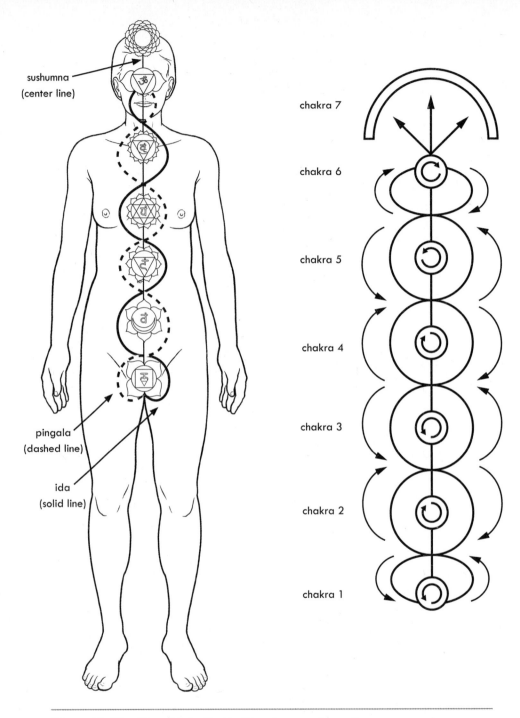

sushumna
(center line)

pingala
(dashed line)

ida
(solid line)

chakra 7

chakra 6

chakra 5

chakra 4

chakra 3

chakra 2

chakra 1

Figure 10: The Three Main Nadis. The three main nadis represent the nervous system of the body. They interact with the seven in-body chakras (right), and when they are balanced, they assist you with being stress free.

EXERCISE 53:
ALIGN YOUR KINETIC CHAIN WITH THE NADIS

In chapter 6 I shared two versions of the kinetic chain. Let's say your performance is underway and you slip out of form. You can quickly realign your kinetic chain, as well as coordinate the cardinal planes and axes, by using the streams to align the nadis. As I explained in chapter 3, the nadis are one set of subtle energy channels. These generally equate with the nerves.

There are three major nadis. As depicted in figure 10, these are as follows:

The Sushumna. This is the main nadi and is the equivalent of the physical spine. Like the chakras, it contains three types of light, shaped like funnels and nested inside each other. The innermost layer is formed of absolute light; the middle layer contains virtual light; and the outermost area is composed of polarity light, or "regular" energy. The spine is the major axis of the body and goes through all the chakras; the vagus nerve also interconnects through the spine.

The Ida. The ida originates at the left side of the first chakra and relates to the right hemisphere of the brain. This means it serves the introverted, the feminine, and the parasympathetic nervous system. This is the relaxing side of the autonomic nervous system.

The Pingala. This nadi emanates from the right side of the first chakra and corresponds to the left hemisphere of the brain, therefore embodying the masculine and active aspects of the body. It also personifies the sympathetic nervous system, or the active and excitatory autonomic nervous system.

To quickly reposition your kinetic chain, conduct Sports Spirit and then request the streams. Ask that they instantaneously flush and clean all three nadis and then perfectly balance them. By doing this, you've established a clear relationship between your ida, pingala, and sushumna and all segments of the body.

EXERCISE 54: ELEMENTAL BOOSTS

One of the ways to best support yourself through game day performance is to pull in the subtle elements that are most vital to your sport. The activity for accessing one or more subtle elements is super easy—you've already been performing it. Simply do the following:

Conduct Sports Spirit.

Request the streams.

Allow these streams to activate and shape the required subtle elements so you can perform a task.

The key is to grasp which subtle elements are most useful for you, depending on your sport, and when to call on the various elements. To help you figure it out, I've created a chart, "Subtle Elements for Various Sports," starting on page 199. Different sports require different elements for distinct purposes, as you can see.

For instance, imagine that you are a soccer player and you're just starting your game. In chapter 6, we discussed the need to create force via the ground (or another material or substance that serves the same purpose), which enables you to create enough force to swim, jump, leap, spring, kick, hit, or whatever. As I shared in that chapter, you can employ a subtle element, not only a physical substance, to build power. Hence, a soccer player can allow the streams to formulate a stronger body of earth energy underneath them in order to create more punch.

Now it's time for our soccer player to move quickly—to get to that ball before someone else does. Sound is the element of power. Here it comes through the streams into the skin and bones to create quick movement. Metal, which can operate like quicksilver, is highly conductive and can add more energy, even as it deflects negativity—like that coming from members of another team.

Need to create a better kinetic chain? More flow? The element of wood provides flexibility, and a soccer player must have that. Fire contributes boosts of energy, which add up to flexibility for spontaneous mechanical actions. What elements can aid a soccer player in remaining positive? Ether is the void. It can eliminate negative thoughts and keep you in the moment, even while the metal element will assist in rejecting negativity and transmitting clarity.

How do the suggested elements stack up for a martial art? Earth, as a solid foundation, strengthens the body and allows you to move off the forces of the ground. It allows you to grapple, throw, be centered, let gravity work for you, and be stabilized. The fire element provides quick boosts of energy for speed. It is dynamic and relentless and allows you to release the heavy power of earth so you can leap and lunge. By combining water, metal, and wood for your mechanics, you are (respectively) inviting circular motion and fluidity and assisting with counter-throwing; operating with an unyielding strength and focus, even as you deflect others' chops, cuts, or smashes (while you yourself remain able to swiftly chop, cut, or smash); and assuring flexibility for gripping, torquing, and more. Assuring positivity with ether is equally vital, for ether represents higher consciousness. In many Eastern systems, this is the non-energy of the void, the space of clearing out your own negativity to achieve samadhi.

What if your sport doesn't show up on the list? Search for a comparable sport. Ice skating is like skiing. Rugby is similar to football. Lacrosse is often considered most comparable to basketball. Hockey is like skiing, as is a version of hockey called bandy.

Softball equates with baseball, while racquetball, badminton, and squash are like tennis. Kayaking and canoeing are adjacent to swimming, although you are separating yourself from the water with another material (the boat). Surfing is actually a lot like skiing, although the water isn't frozen. I would put wrestling into the martial arts category and snowboarding into skiing. Basically, consider what types of movements and interactions with the environment are required for your sport in order to place it on the following chart. However, make any elemental changes you believe are necessary.

For instance, gymnastics is quite similar to skiing; however, the medium is the air. Hence, you might change your grounding element from water and ether to air plus the grounding element you most often use. If you perform on the bars or balance beam, that element might be wood. If you use the mat, you could use stone or earth.

Subtle Elements for Various Sports

Sport	Grounding Element	Speed Element	Mechanics Element	Positivity Element
Baseball	Star and Earth	Fire	Light and Wood	Ether and Metal
Basketball	Stone	Fire and Metal (like quicksilver)	Water	Light
Bicycling	Earth or Stone and Air	Air	Metal (like quicksilver)	Ether

Sport	Grounding Element	Speed Element	Mechanics Element	Positivity Element
Football	Earth	Fire and Metal (like quicksilver)	Stone and Fire	Star and Metal
Golf	Earth	Air	Wood	Light
Martial Arts	Earth	Fire	Water, Metal, Wood	Ether
Running/Hiking/ Walking	Earth and Air	Air	Sound	Light
Skiing	Water and Ether	Fire	Water	Light
Soccer	Earth	Sound and Metal (like quicksilver)	Fire and Wood	Ether and Metal
Swimming	Water	Air	Light	Sound
Tennis	Stone	Air	Stone and Fire	Air
Volleyball	Stone	Fire	Air	Sound

Post–Game Day

You've done it! You have performed on your game day. There are a few subtle activities that can be very useful afterward. These are listed in the order of what to do, from closest to your performance (same day) to further away (within two to three days).

Congratulate yourself. It's important to praise yourself for whatever worked out great. For now, ignore the negatives. You must be your own cheerleader. If you're a coach, focus on the positives for your athlete.

Return to your center of gravity. You know how to do this by now. Either reaffirm Gamma Gameline or enter that state, and then balance yourself physically with your center of gravity subtly linked to your strongest chakra center.

Focus on your breathing. Breathe deeply and, while doing so, ask for the streams to run through your body in order to release you from any mental or physical toxins or aftermath. These streams can also begin to rebuild and restore your muscles and other tissues, so you can also request that the appropriate subtle elements enter via the streams for that purpose.

Assess performance with a trusted friend or coach. You can also use a member of your invisible board of directors. Examine the upsides and the downsides of your performance, and if you need to make changes to your mental game, mechanics, or anything else, insert those changes into your preparation plan.

Select any vibrational remedies that might be useful. I've indicated a few that are really terrific for post–game day in the next section, "Vibrational Remedies for Performance."

Celebrate. What does that mean to you? Not an entire chocolate cake, I hope, but maybe a slice! Some athletes celebrate by conducting a heavy-duty workout afterward. That's optional.

Vibrational Remedies for Performance

There are a lot of Bach Flower Essences that can be useful both pre- and post-performance and even during (if applicable). I'll list those and provide a few tips next.

Cherry Plum: Addresses fear of losing control and appearing foolish. Good remedy for performance anxiety or if you feel like you blew an aspect of your game day.

Elm: For loss of confidence. To use any time around game day, especially during performance if your confidence starts to slide.

Gentian: To use when things are going wrong. Wonderful remedy to employ during performance and afterward if you believe you made mistakes.

Holly: For negative feelings aggressively directed toward others. Are you too angry at your competition? Try holly. Are others really negative toward you? Go for holly.

Hornbeam: If you feel exhausted before making an effort, hornbeam will help you cope. Best for pre-game.

Mimulus: Relieves known fears. Can be used anytime in relation to performance. Helpful in post-performance to deal with the results of having been imperfect.

Oak: To stay steady under pressure. Use before or during performance.

Olive: For exhaustion after an effort. Great for post–game day.

Pine: Good if you're blaming yourself or others for things that were done or not done. Perfect antidote if you are feeling negative post-game.

Rock Rose: Buffers against terror. Terrific for pre–game day jitters.

Star of Bethlehem: For aftereffects of shock. If your game went really well or really poorly, try this remedy.

Sweet Chestnut: When you've reached your limits and just don't think you can keep going, before or during a game, use this remedy.

Walnut: Provides protection against outside influences, especially useful before and during game day.

White Chestnut: Bolsters against unwanted thoughts and mental arguments. Really, employ this one anytime!

Willow: Reduces resentments. Do you sense you've been slighted or cheated? Try willow.

In the end, an athlete is always working toward a performance; so is the coach assisting the athlete. In this chapter, we covered the subtle basics of pre-, during, and post-game day. You learned lots of exercises, a way to apply the subtle elements, and vibrational remedies to make that day a great one.

Next we're going to look at an incredibly vital aspect of sports: the psychological game.

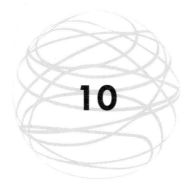

10

Dealing with Ups and Downs

I need this. I need to see other amazing people fall apart.

—Chloe Kim, snowboarding gold medalist,
on getting okay with her ups and downs

There are two well-known quotes that serve as the foundation for this chapter. They are seemingly opposite, but that's on purpose because they are both equally true.

The first speaks to perseverance in the face of so-called failure and was uttered by basketball star Michael Jordan, who first stated it in a Nike commercial and then discussed it in a *Chicago Tribune* article in 1997: "I've missed more than 9,000 shots in my career. I've lost almost 300 games ... I've failed over and over and over again in my life. And that is why I succeed."[51]

The other vital statement was shared with the world by gymnast Simone Biles, considered the greatest female gymnast of all time, upon withdrawing from key events at the 2021 Tokyo Olympics to care for her mental health. Said Biles, "We have to focus on ourselves because at the end of the day, we're human, too. We have to protect our mind and our body rather than just go out there and do what the world wants us to do."[52]

Though these two statements seem to point in opposite directions, they can be bridged. The bridging of these viewpoints is the key to your true success as an athlete, whether you

51   Zorn, "Without Failure, Jordan Would Be a False Idol."
52   Lies and Tetrault-Farber, "Simone Biles Says Gymnastics Is Not Everything."

are of the everyday variety or among the elite in your sport. It also largely determines how you can most thoroughly embody your soul in what is a very human and imperfect body.

Michael Jordan's statement implies that athletic success is a matter of physical perseverance, perhaps to the point of ignoring the flailing mind: no matter the cost, gut it out. What happens when we do this, when we compartmentalize our sense of failure to push through to the other side? Simone Biles's admission is that sometimes true courage involves stepping back from the precipice to take time to tend the stressed-out mind. Her attitude shows that the edges of life blur—and that athletic decisions must be gauged according to a formula of an interdependent body, mind, and soul.

Biles's actions at the Olympics also ushered her into a small but emerging club of athletes who have been touting the importance of mental health. If the mind suffers, so does the body. For decades, athletics have really been just an extension of a militaristic mindset: set the goal and then muscle through, no matter the cost. Obey your chain of command. Don't be needy.

Is it time to override the old-fashioned perception that saying "I cannot" is a weakness? I believe it is.

The truth is that when it comes to a sport, some days, weeks, and even years are terrific. Then there are the times that aren't, and they can get really dark. That's because a sport isn't just a physical endeavor. It is also a psychological one.

Almost every athlete I've met has spent time on the downward spiral. Some hit bottom relatively quickly and can start climbing back up at a reasonable pace. Some step out of their sport altogether, unable to cope physically or mentally. Yet others go "one step backward, two steps forward" with a lot of emotional and maybe even physical pain.

How do you negotiate the so-called negative feelings associated with so many aspects of athletics? How do you support all parts of yourself in a loving, rather than judgmental, way?

Well, the purpose of this chapter isn't to help you erase your emotions or mental struggles. These are a real part of life, especially of the sports world. But I will provide perspectives and exercises aimed at helping you deal with downer feelings and thoughts, and maybe even transform your experience through the rough times.

I've already introduced many techniques that can alleviate challenging emotional issues. Gamma Gameline can support you in centering yourself and clearing subconscious beliefs. EFT empowers you to create positive affirmations. Performing an energy analysis and healing can help you release harmful forces. But now it's time for some new ideas, which range from deconstructing emotions to activating the various "molecules of joy" produced in a healthy body. Want something different or something more? How about clearing others' energies from your own energy field or employing beneficial essential oils? In the end, no matter what activities you are attracted to, know one thing: people care about you, so care about yourself.

When you're struggling, you need to keep your world small enough that you are protected from naysayers. Think of the courage it took for Biles to stand up against the entire world in order to focus on the coaches, teammates, friends, and family members who cared more about her than about her appearance at a performance.

At the same time, you want to stretch your world so that it is large enough for you to have time for love and peace. Know that every athlete undergoes at least one dark night of the soul, and know that if you're in yours, there really is a new dawn on the other side. Love yourself enough to look for that light, and be gentle with the process.

The Dark Night of the Soul

It's easy to get pulled down the river and over a waterfall, and athletes are especially prone to a sudden slide. The pressures of a sport are compounded by the idea that if you just keep pushing physically while stuffing your thoughts and emotions into a box, you'll get through. And to complicate matters further, sports can be all consuming, often determining one's identity, and this is true of both ordinary and professional athletes.

I saw my son, Gabriel, go through this in the most painful of ways.

The most challenging time in his college baseball year occurred after he was struck with COVID-19. He endured the typical flu-like physical symptoms, but then the virus settled into his lower back. Standing on the pitching mound, he never knew whether his back was going to obey his brain and let him pitch or if his body would simply freeze up and he wouldn't be able to move at all. The lack of physical control made him so nervous he didn't even want to step onto that mound.

His coaches were of little help. They didn't understand either the physical or mental hardships he was facing. One of the coaches implied he should just push through it. Another said he cared about what Gabe was going through but couldn't help him readjust his mechanics or otherwise support him in getting his lost mojo back. A few teammates implied that he was making it all up. They even seemed pleased with his struggles, perhaps out of jealousy; before his back problems, Gabe had been a top draft pick. Eventually, the draft turned elusive and then disappeared, as his stats weren't there anymore.

Gabe's world narrowed to a few supporters. The physical stress was overwhelming, matched by the emotional frustration and the mental challenges of making new life- and sports-based decisions. Should he quit ball altogether? Or should he just quit his current team and look for a new college to play for? If he did that, would another school even want him?

Gabe didn't only hit one bottom; he hit several. So did the people who cared about him. I found myself empathically going through many of his feelings, frequently tearing up. Even though I was only a mom in the bleachers, I had to put many of the tools in this chapter to work to keep myself strong enough to be a supportive figure and help him negotiate his decisions each step of the way. Even then, I failed him in one regard.

At one point, Gabe wanted to withdraw from his school and focus on training. Every male advisor told him this was a mistake. I thought it was smart, but old-school thinking about sports overrode his needs and both of our opinions: "No one will want you again if you put yourself first. You'll be known as a quitter."

If only we had been able to witness Simone Biles granting herself grace *before* this happened to Gabe instead of after.

If only we had already seen tennis player Naomi Osaka refuse to participate in a press conference at Roland Garros because it would impact her negatively, and then withdraw from the French Open to preserve her mental health. As she said in an article she penned for *Time*, "There can be moments for any of us when we are dealing with issues behind the scenes."[53]

If only we had recognized the courage that had already been demonstrated by basketball stars like Kyrie Irving, DeMar DeRozan, and Kevin Love, who spoke openly about mental health challenges.

The militaristic aspect of sports insisted that Gabe compartmentalize his stress—that he ignore his body's weakness and his mind's doubts and force himself forward. Knowing what I now know, I say, "Really?" In fact, many of the tools in this chapter are designed to give you a way through that doesn't call for force of will but rather for gently stepping through your decisions.

In the end, Gabe decided to trust his innate abilities and leave the school, which had nothing to give him. Even then, he shared that it was going to be hard to tell them he was

---

53   Osaka, "Naomi Osaka: 'It's O.K. Not to Be O.K.'"

quitting. "It's like a bad relationship, Mom," he admitted. "You feel so bad about yourself that you don't think you deserve better."

Then Gabe asked me for a psychic sign to indicate that his decision would be helpful.

The morning he made that request, I pulled out of a gas station to drive to a game. Right in front of me was a truck. Spread across the entire back window was a single word: "Gabriel."

And the license plate? It contained letters meaning the equivalent of "1Yes" and "Hero"—or, be a hero in your own life and put yourself first.

After he gave notice at his school, Gabe went to Seattle to train. Within a week, his mechanics and his power were back. He called me with a simple message: "I believe in energy."

The team had simply become so negative (except for a few teammates and one of the coaches, who wished him well when he left) that Gabe hadn't even been able to see himself as a baseball player anymore. He needed a new environment.

And with that new environment, everything changed. Not just his pitching, which by the end of the summer was more than back on track—well into the mid-90s in terms of velocity, in fact. But also, almost right after leaving the school, he received several full-ride and partial scholarship offers. He perused those options carefully. He wanted positive coaches who communicated well and were committed to getting him drafted. He selected the school that invested the time to look at all his films closely and let him know they could have assisted him through the crisis.

Gabe's situation reveals the impact of negative athletic performance on the body as well as the mind and, in general, on your perceptions of life. But the opposite situation can be just as hard: the hardships of life can affect your sport.

At the same time as Gabe's situation was unfolding, I was helping a cross-country skier client. She loved that form of skiing, and especially competing in the annual Birkebeiner, the longest cross-country ski race in North America. She never placed high in it, but it didn't matter: the Birkebeiner was her deal. Then getting divorced forced her back into a job that gave her no time off.

My client missed two annual Birkebeiner events and had very little time for her beloved cross-country skiing. She became seriously depressed—and actually lost interest in life. When the third Birkebeiner came up with enough time for her to enter, she passed on it anyway. She didn't see the point. She hadn't been training, and she knew she'd be a failure compared to her previous self. She didn't want to embarrass herself. Lacking a place in her life for her sport, her emotions spiraled even further, until she saw a psychiatrist for clinical depression.

My client never did return to the Birkebeiner. She didn't see, realistically, how to readjust her life to train hard enough for it. After grieving, however, she found a way to return to her beloved sport. She joined a cross-country ski club. The result? She made a lot of new friends and her mood picked up. She also started using the gym at her place of business to create some of the chemicals of joy that athletes get when they are exercising—and I'll cover those further along in this chapter.

Why is a sport so intertwined with all other levels of well-being?

First off, athletics is body-based, and the body is an instrument that changes daily, even more so as we age, and especially when we are emotionally stressed or physically injured. As well, the very nature of competition can invoke or stir latent psychological issues. Everyone has childhood issues, as well as inherited ancestral memories, and these are easily triggered under stress. Indeed, some athletes are prone to various emotional tendencies, which can either help or hurt.

Think about obsessive-compulsive disorder (OCD). Technically, one facet of OCD is an adherence to perfectionism. I've devoted quite a bit of ink in this book to discussing the dangers of overboard perfectionism. But athletes, especially elite ones, have to get their game on. To beat the competition, you have to be better than others. You need a smarter or harder workout program, better coaching, or insanely high-end sports gear and tech. And what about those mechanics? If an athlete starts to slide or is just plain tired, it's easy for OCD-like attributes to take off, creating suffering in the mind and heart.

Next, think about the bells and whistles—and highlights and lowlights—that often accompany a sport. Especially at the competitive level, athletes often have to deal with bullying and possibly even eating issues, depression, or anxiety caused by pressure. Then there is the tendency to over-train or lose sleep. How about the temptation to dope or take other unhealthy shortcuts?

What about life's deeper issues, like gender identity? It is incredibly sad that the first active NFL football player who came out as gay did that in 2021. Kudos to Carl Nassib. What a "tell" about the militaristic nature of sports, however. How long must we endure the philosophy that an athlete isn't supposed to be who they really are?

As I shared in chapter 7, the serious or even everyday athlete might also be affected by money stressors. Maybe your thing is hiking. You'd love to take that world-famous trek, but you can't afford it, so … maybe not.

Sometimes lower economic status makes certain athletes take unnatural risks. I remember visiting with a parent from a Texas team when I was down in Jupiter, Florida, for a baseball competition. The father of a player pointed to a young Hispanic team member and shared how sad he felt because many of the southern club teams—youth teams operated independently of the school system—often let in really young immigrant kids who simply wanted a chance. He said a lot of the MLB teams recruited these kids for pennies on the dollar, figuring that for every hundred they brought in, they might get one good one worth keeping. The rest of them would be spit out of the machine a year or two later, at a very young age, with no education or real job opportunities.

If you were in that position, maybe you'd take a chance anyway, right?

In general, I've learned that internally motivated athletes have a better chance of coping with the ups and downs of their sport than do externally motivated ones. Many an athlete I've worked with quits their sport when they can't please their parent or coach or suffers more torment when things go wrong than internally driven performers do. I'm good with athletes who quit a sport or change how they do it. In all these and infinite other sports scenarios, however, the mental and emotional anguish is very real, and it is only compounded by the fact that not only are athletes affected by unnatural expectations, but they are influenced by others' energies as well.

Think of it. Gabe only started to *really* believe in the effects of others' energies after the team's negativity further deteriorated his performance. It was at that point that he decided his main criterion for selecting a new school had to be the nature of the energetic environment.

In light of that truth—and the fact that so few mind-body experts deal with this aspect of subtle energy—I'm going to delve deeper into the issue of others' energies, offering a related exercise.

Taking on Others' Energies

Marco had been an Olympian athlete for Cuba, scoring a bronze medal in his sport. Then, joining others on a group of rafts, he undertook the treacherous journey across the waters from Cuba to the United States. Nearly everyone else died in the water; he watched as many fell to sharks. After a few years in America, he obtained residency, but that wasn't the end of his problems.

He put his sport to work and offered lessons in it. (To protect his privacy, I won't mention the sport.) But the horrors of the journey out of Cuba, as well as survivor's guilt, took a toll, and he became addicted to crack.

I met Marco when he had just come out of his third rehab center. He was starting to give lessons in his sport again. I paid for a set of lessons and then didn't hear from him for a while—until he called from a psychiatric ward. He told me that he couldn't help it: money burned a hole in his pocket, he said, so he had gone on the street to buy crack. Then he told me something he was afraid to tell his counselors.

"When I'm on crack, I'm in darkness." He added, "And then dark spirits whisper to me. They tell me I'm worthless and that I should end it all."

In fact, the police had found Marco on a cliff getting ready to jump in response to the voices. Hence, the lockup in the psych ward.

Off and on over the years, I stayed in touch with Marco. At one point he committed a crime and ended up in jail. There he got help from a therapist who, interestingly, specialized in exorcisms. Now free of the darkness, Marco is living clean and simply, and teaching again.

I'm not making the point that when athletes are in the dumps, they are all subjected to entities or forces. I am saying, however, that when someone is down, their internal issues arise. Plus, new ones can develop, creating a vulnerability to taking on others' energies—and even becoming susceptible to entities. Because of this, before you seek to work on your issues, I suggest you use the following exercise to free yourself from what is not your own.

EXERCISE 55:
FREEING YOURSELF FROM OTHERS' ENERGIES

This simple exercise can help release you from energy that is not yours.

Walk through Sports Spirit and then request the streams. Ask guidance to activate your intuition so you can receive a response to these questions:

- ▸ What percentage of the distress I'm going through is mine?
- ▸ What percentage comes from others?

Spend some time getting a better sense of your own challenges. You can always use exercise 15, Energy Analysis and Healing, to work on these issues, and you can employ additional exercises found in this chapter. Then request that the streams carry from you all energies that are not your own. Know that cords and holds will be disintegrated, and all earthly and otherworldly sources will be assessed. These released energies will be returned to their original source in a safe way, if appropriate, or dealt with in a kind and loving manner. Ask for additional streams to plug holes that are now in your system and activate your own vital spirit, and then, when you're ready, return to your day.

Healing Your Emotions

Emotions are a vital part of all sports. They motivate, drive, encourage, and indicate when it's time to rest and recover. But they can also cost energy and peace of mind and create suffering.

Often, an athletic problem brings up hard emotions. As a case in point, medicine is finally examining the effects of head injuries on athletes, specifically by studying the progressive degeneration of all faculties that is suffered at the hands of chronic traumatic encephalopathy (CTE)—also known as a concussion. Out-of-control emotions are standard in CTE victims. But emotions also negatively affect sports performance. Either way, we have to deal with emotions intruding on our enjoyment of a sport or of life itself.

In chapter 9 I showed you how to transform intrusive feelings and awarenesses. In this section you're going to work more directly on any emotions that are impeding your athletic joy. Basically, I'll show you how to deconstruct an emotion that is inhibitory or harmful so you can analyze its separate components and grow from this understanding.

That's right: I said "components" of an emotion. There are two constituents of any emotion: at least one feeling and at least one belief that have become fused together.

Think about it. Feelings are messages from the body. They speak a language we need to heed. While no feeling is inherently good or bad, there are helpful and unhelpful responses to feelings. As I'll discuss later in this chapter, the emotion of anger insists that you need to set a boundary. If you establish a boundary by speaking politely or walking away, you won't cause harm to yourself or others. A less useful response to someone who is offending you would be to throw your hamburger in their face. That won't get you anywhere; at the very least, you'll look like a jerk. Worse, what if you violently shoved a medicine ball onto a workout mate who offended you? You could end up in jail.

Beliefs are the rungs of the ladder to decision making. Our beliefs get us where we want to go. For an athlete, beliefs are all-important. If you believe you can improve your mechanics, you are much more likely to do so. If you don't think you can do it, you probably won't.

Beliefs are made of thoughts. By themselves, thoughts are merely opinions. The thought *I am stupid* is not a fact; it is an opinion. Most of our beliefs are actually opinions gone wrong. In fact, according to the National Science Foundation, the typical person has between 12,000 and 60,000 thoughts a day. Of these, 80 percent are negative, and 95 percent of these negative thoughts are repetitive.[54]

In general, most of our thoughts are like dust bunnies—sometimes more like dust tornadoes—that create negative drama in our minds. Worse, we usually believe all those negative thoughts are true. In turn, we act from these unhealthy beliefs.

Most of our beliefs really are of the dust bunny variety. They are empty and silly. Underneath all of these, however, are fundamental beliefs, most of which are actually lies. These are very destructive. In fact, there are six major types of negative beliefs that you'll learn about in the related exercise. One of these is the belief that you are worthless. If believing yourself worthless underlies thousands of sub-beliefs, think about how impossible it might be to become really good at your sport or be happy executing it. It's extremely hard to change one of these six potent core beliefs when it is bonded with a feeling.

One key is to understand why feelings and beliefs so often partner—and fail to get divorced, although the relationship is strained at best.

Fundamentally, we construct emotions because our brain can then bypass the need to make the same decisions over and over again. It's far easier to live life on automatic than it is to tediously heed every feeling or think through every single thought.

For example, think about the association that most of us make when a bee is buzzing around our body. The feeling is fear, and the thought might be *That bee can hurt me.* When a bee is really close, you don't have time to feel that fear and figure out what it means while also analyzing the idea that a bee can sting. The fear and thought have already bonded to make you move so you don't get stung.

Athletes depend on emotions. If you're biking down a mountain and a truck roars up behind you, you had better be scared and know that you could get hit. The instantaneous

---

54   Verma, "Destroy Negativity from Your Mind."

swerve of your handlebars might save your life. But emotions that have no usefulness? Not a good thing.

For instance, imagine that you are undergoing a downward spiral caused by a physical injury, but you don't realize that an emotional reaction is rearing its head. Here comes that fear of failure, along with the subconscious belief *No one ever recovers fully from injury.* Your mood gets worse and worse, the fear grows, and you walk around with a pit in your stomach all the time. Your body tenses, and it becomes harder and harder to actually recover.

The emotion becomes a predictor of outcome.

It's vital to pay attention to your feelings and honor their innate message. It's also important to alter destructive beliefs and change them into constructive ones. The following four-part exercise will help you do just that.

EXERCISE 56: HEALING YOUR EMOTIONS

Step One: Embrace the Emotion. Aware of a harmful emotion? Enter a meditative state and conduct Sports Spirit. Ask guidance to provide streams for clarity; they will also activate your intuition. Then focus on the challenging emotion.

- ▸ Where is it in your body?
- ▸ How is it affecting you?
- ▸ When or how did it start?

Seek to understand the emotion until you become aware of the major feeling that lies within it. The feeling will be sadness, fear, anger, disgust, or even joy. Set that feeling aside for a moment; you will deal with it in step two.

Now request that the streams help you determine the major destructive belief. Remember: it will be a lie, although it might seem to be true. Nonetheless, no matter what, it will be negative and shaming. Also put this belief aside. You will do further work with it in step three.

Step Two: Mature the Feeling. You are aware of the main feeling associated with the harsh emotion. The good news is that there is a message in every one of the five major feeling constellations. Read through the following to highlight this truth.

Feeling Constellation	Meaning
Sadness	Love. Love seems to be missing; I must uncover the love that is there or find another source.
Fear	Safety. I'm not safe and I need to change direction to become safe.
Anger	Boundaries. There has been a boundary violation, and I must establish a new boundary.
Disgust	Yuck. This is not good for me, and I need to stop or get rid of something.
Joy	Yes. I want more of the same.

Once you've determined the message of the feeling, use your intuition to "talk" with the feeling, asking it questions like these:

How can I obey your suggestion?

What do I need to do differently to gain what you are offering?

Now focus on this key:

All feelings, if you pay attention to their messages and perform any activities needed to make good on them, will eventually transform or mature into a version of joy.

That's right. All feelings will eventually lead to joy.

For instance, imagine that you're sad because you are injured and aren't going to be able to perform for a year. Sadness is about love. How can sitting on a bench—or at home—make you feel more love?

Well, you can decide to do self-care or take up a new hobby. By choosing such a path of love, a form of joy will eventually emerge, such as appreciation, self-compassion, or patience.

Now let's imagine that a coach is disrespectful toward you. Why wouldn't you feel angry in that situation? The job of anger is to make you establish a perimeter. That doesn't mean you hit the coach on the head or try to get them fired. (And good luck with that, anyway.) Maybe instead you decide that your coach's attitude doesn't need to determine your self-esteem or that you'll change your situation and find a different coach. In the end, the resulting joy might come in the form of relief, pride, or increased determination.

Once you've finished maturing the feeling, which can take some time, move on to step three.

Step Three: Shift the Belief. All beliefs or opinions can be organized into seven primary categories, with every negative or dysfunctional belief in opposition to a correlating positive and correct belief. Look through this list to focus on the negative belief that best represents the one you came to in step one.

Positive/Truth	Negative/Lie
I am worthy	I am worthless
I am good	I am evil
I am lovable	I am unlovable
I am deserving	I am undeserving
I am powerful	I am powerless
I have value	I have no value
I am connected	I am separate

At this point, it's important to decide to switch the negative belief for its truthful counterpart. Anchor into the lie. Get a sense of how it makes you feel about yourself, your needs, and your ability as an athlete. Then decide. *Decide* that this belief is a lie. It is a false opinion. It is not true. To make good on this decision, request that the streams you summoned in step one—or new ones you may call for aid—replace the wrong idea with the correct one. As you move back into your life, you'll want to keep reiterating that thought consciously.

Step Four: Celebrate! You've separated a matched feeling and belief. That feeling is now free to be continually matured, and the negative belief has been altered into a true one. *Yeah!* How can you reward yourself? Do something special, then keep working with this exercise as needed.

If you need to shift an emotion on a dime, at least temporarily, use the following add-on exercise.

EXERCISE 57: CENTER IN YOUR SPINE

As you'll recall, in chapter 6 we discussed energetic anxiety and depression. If your soul or your awareness is too far in front of a chakra in relation to the spine, you can become energetically anxious. If it's too far back, you can feel energetically depressed.

When you're aware of an emotional imbalance, immediately conduct Sports Spirit and request that the streams align your soul and awareness in the center of each chakra and the spine. You'll now be more self-contained and calm. Do this as often as required, at least until you have time to deep-dive the issues.

Molecules of Joy

There are at least seven molecules of joy that need to be active for you to feel ease and comfort as well as feel energized when it's push time.

Most individuals are constantly seeking, albeit unconsciously, to materialize these molecules, which are neurotransmitters mainly produced by endocrine glands. The problem is that we often stimulate their release in unhealthy ways.

We can become too dependent on cannabis (as we can on any substance!) or exercise too much in order to stimulate our natural endocannabinoids. We employ alcohol to calm our adrenals, which are often overworked. And who wouldn't agree that cocaine, sugar, or other crazy reward mechanisms are poor substitutes for healthy ways to increase our dopamine?

When we're in a funk, there are a lot of activities that can stimulate the production of our seven major joy molecules. Most important for our discussion, there are subtle mechanisms that can improve matters too, which I'll now emphasize.

Note: For additional tips about these molecules related specifically to sports, I suggest reading Christopher Bergland's book *The Athlete's Way*. Most of the labels I've given to these seven joy molecules come from Bergland.

Endocannabinoids: Bliss Molecules

Networked throughout the body is a "cannabis" system that is partially responsible for moments of bliss. Yup—the body produces neurochemicals similar to those in marijuana, or cannabis. So you can better understand your happiness-making chemicals, the overall system that creates these bliss molecules is called the endocannabinoid system, and it is composed of cannabinoid receptors, endocannabinoids (the neurochemicals), and specialized enzymes.

These neurochemicals and their cellular receptors are found throughout the body, including in the brain, connective tissue, glands, and immune cells. The system in its entirety is quite busy bringing balance and cheer to all parts of the body. As well, these molecules can be found at the sites of injuries, where they prevent excessive nerve firing and help prevent inflammation. They also mediate our relationship with the external environment and promote humor, creativity, and joy.[55] Problems with this system can lead to all sorts of issues, among them anxiety, depression, and digestive challenges.[56]

So how do you help your body balance its endocannabinoid system? First, work with a professional to make sure that any physical approaches will be helpful and beneficial. But no matter what, consider the subtle actions you can take.

PHYSICAL BALANCE. Try herbs like black pepper, cloves, hops, and lemon balm. Eat foods high in omega-3 fatty acids, like fish and hemp and chia seeds. Also do high-aerobics exercises, if your body isn't already burned out from too much exercise.[57]

SUBTLE BALANCE. Subtle energetics afford us the luxury of utilizing a plant even if we don't know which one to take or can't find or can't process one we think might work. This exercise comes from a form of plant medicine that I have studied in many places around the world.

All the shamans I've met find that the easiest ways to incorporate the energy of a plant is to call upon the spirit of that plant. That way you don't actually have to use the plant's physical properties; you can simply bring in its subtle energies. In other words, you don't have to smoke or ingest cannabis. Rather, use the following short process to call upon the spirit of cannabis to aid you.

After going through Sports Spirit, ask guidance to connect you with the spirit or essence of the cannabis plant. Rest in a meditative state with this consciousness for a few minutes, and then request that the streams be made available to carry the properties of that plant into you. These streams will continue to provide ease and calm.

Dopamine: Reward Molecules

When we accomplish something, our body manufactures dopamine to give us that rush of reward for our efforts. This neurotransmitter is all about pleasure, even as it keeps your nerve cells happily communicating. In fact, dopamine runs many physical systems while also helping your body process pain. However, too much or too little dopamine in your system is linked to several mental and emotional disorders, such as schizophrenia, attention deficit hyperactivity disorder (ADHD), and various addictions.[58]

---

55   Sulak, "Introduction to the Endocannabinoid System."
56   Cibdol, "How to Balance Your Endocannabinoid System."
57   Ibid.
58   Cristol, "What Is Dopamine?"

Having enough dopamine not only gives us that *Yeah, we did it!* but also helps us deal with stress. Recent scientific studies are showing that elite athletes might also differ from nonprofessional ones in that the elites are genetically equipped with the ability to transport more dopamine.[59]

You can increase your dopamine levels by exercising, but what happens when you're down and out? What if you're injured or can't grab time to exercise, much like my cross-country skiing client I discussed at the beginning of this chapter? What if you're frozen out of your sport, short term or long term? What if you're undergoing the depths of a spiral and what used to bring you pleasure, including being noticed or respected, has tanked?

Consider boosting low dopamine levels in these ways.

PHYSICAL BALANCE. Exercise in whatever way is practical and get enough protein (specifically tyrosine, one of the amino acids that make dopamine). Make sure to get enough sleep. When you can, listen to music and get some sun—safely.

SUBTLE BALANCE. Try your hand at these subtle energy ideas:

For one, it's been found that performing one hour of yoga six days a week increases dopamine levels, whereas undergoing a thirty-minute session of treadmill running does not. Clearing your mind through meditating for one hour has also been shown to greatly increase dopamine production, at least in experienced meditation teachers.[60] Then start rewarding yourself for non-athletic practices. Draw a picture and put it on your refrigerator. Really! Volunteer somewhere that makes you feel good about your participation. In general, look to Eastern care modalities and creative and loving activities to get out of a funk.

Oxytocin: Bonding Molecules

When love is in the air, our body naturally produces more oxytocin, and sometimes in men a molecule called vasopressin, a kissing cousin. Mainly made in the hypothalamus and secreted by the pituitary, this important hormone is also produced in the heart.

When we're in a close relationship or are part of a supportive group such as a team or a family, we're most likely to be producing enough of this bonding hormone, which creates feelings of comfort and ease. But what if we aren't experiencing a lot of love? If our athletic team members aren't supportive? We experience a resulting reduction of oxytocin, and in comes the sense of being alone. Now it's far easier to spiral downward.

---

59   Wylie, "Olympic Gold May Depend on the Brain's Reward Chemical."
60   Julson, "10 Best Ways to Increase Dopamine Levels Naturally."

For example, I once worked with a former professional baseball pitcher who had never recovered from Tommy John elbow surgery. He believes that the real cause wasn't insufficient recovery; rather, it was that his teammates didn't want him to succeed.

How can you boost up your oxytocin levels when you're lacking it? How can you start to feel lovable again, an important factor in dealing with the ups and downs of a sport? The key is to connect, and here are some ideas.

PHYSICAL BALANCE. Get skin-physical. Hug, cuddle. Get a dog or borrow someone else's and take it for a walk. Go for massages or do other types of body care. Create your short list of those people who are proving that they are really there for you and spend time with them, in person or on the phone. Forget the others for now.

SUBTLE BALANCE. Mainly, I recommend working simultaneously with your fourth and sixth chakras.

The fourth chakra is related to the physical heart. That sixth chakra governs the hypothalamus and the pituitary gland. Work with the following meditation to coordinate the activities of oxytocin.

After running through Sports Spirit, bring your focus to the inner wheel of your fourth chakra. Request that guidance activate the absolute light within that space and bring the resulting streams of brilliance throughout your entire physical and subtle systems. Now rest your focus in the center of your sixth chakra. Within, ask that your essence create an image of your true identity. In other words, ask to envision yourself the way your Higher Spirit sees you.

Accept this vision in any way it shows up—as a video, a single picture, or even as colors and shapes. Then let yourself actively feel how your Higher Spirit feels about you.

You are beloved.

Take that in.

Be one with the truth of yourself and who you really are, even as the streams activate and supply you with your needed bonding hormones. Close when you are ready.

Endorphins: Pain-Killing Molecules

When we're in pain or under stress, here come our mini Captain Marvels: the endorphins. Or at least, that's the idea.

These neurotransmitters are generated by the hypothalamus and the pituitary, and there are twenty different types. The most frequently studied among them, called beta-endorphins, actually eliminate pain better than opioids do. When we don't have the appropriate supply of them, however, we might search out negative sources of support; that's what opioid addicts are doing.

Think on it ... the similarity between the words "endorphins" and "morphine," which is the source of many opioids.

Low levels of endorphins can lead to everything from fatigue to depression, as well as aches and pains.

Endorphins are similar to dopamine molecules, and they often work together. The main difference between them is that endorphins, while reducing pain, can also tell the body when to make dopamine. Thus they are busy alleviating pain while your dopamine is picking you up.[61]

Ironically, I find that a lot of athletes experience low endorphins because they have undergone an injury. Exercise is one of the most natural ways to boost the presence of this pain-killing molecule, and when you're injured, it's hard to exercise. Also, depression, such as occurs if you're struggling athletically, can make it harder to move around too. So help yourself in these ways.

PHYSICAL BALANCE. Get some form of exercise. Make sure you do anaerobic cardio and strength training, not just aerobic exercise. Also try yoga, spicy foods, dark chocolate, and laughing.

SUBTLE BALANCE. Needling—the use of acupuncture needles on the meridians—produces endorphins, releasing pain and restoring ease.[62] If you're not into needles, I heartily suggest using EFT, which I introduced you to in chapter 4.

Gamma Aminobutyric Acid (GABA): Anti-Anxiety Molecules

GABA is a neurotransmitter that can block impulses from traveling between the nerve cells in the brain. Figuratively, it keeps them from "talking too much." Too much conversation among them can lead to anxiety or mood disorders.

Some people are low in GABA and don't know it. GABA can plummet when we're experiencing chronic stress, a poor diet, or not enough exercise. When an athlete can't get their workouts or is feeling too much pressure, their GABA levels might fall, leading to crazy

---

61   Good Therapy, "Endorphins."
62   Integrity Women's Health, "Demystifying Acupuncture."

anxiety.[63] Some athletes are so used to being anxious that they don't even know how bad their situation is.

What to do if you think you are low in GABA? See a naturopath or other specialist and consider the following.

PHYSICAL BALANCE. Consider GABA supplements, getting back to exercising more if you've fallen off the wagon, and yoga.

SUBTLE BALANCE. Back in chapter 6 I talked about how important it is to remain centered in the middle of your spine and the center wheels of your chakras. When our soul is too far forward in relation to the central axis, the related chakra is future-forward, and we get energetically anxious: we're too involved in predicting the future. When our soul is too far backward in relation to the central axis, that chakra is historically oriented. We can become energetically depressed, or stuck in the past. And I have found that if we're energetically anxious in one area of our life, we're energetically depressed somewhere else.

One practice is to use the four-six breathing that you learned in exercise 1 several times a day. After conducting Sports Spirit, every time you breathe in, ask for the streams and allow them to center your soul in the middle of the spine and the inner wheel of every chakra. Every time you breathe out, ask that whatever is plaguing you be released.

You can also consistently practice Gamma Gameline, which will continue to align and realign you.

Serotonin: Worthiness Molecules

Serotonin is made in the "head brain" and in the enteric nervous system, or "gut brain." It's a feel-good neurotransmitter, and when we don't have enough of it, it's easy to lose athletic motivation and experience depression. Since melatonin is made in the brain from serotonin, too little serotonin in the brain can also lead to sleep disorders.

The truth is that about 95 percent of your serotonin is made in your gut.[64] Most of my clients with too much serotonin in the gut experience heavy-duty anxiety in the body; often, their serotonin levels are consequently too low in the brain, causing head-based depression. It's essential to balance your serotonin, or you can become afflicted with anything from being overly agitated to depressed to sick in the stomach.

---

63   Purdy, "Is Your High Functioning Anxiety Caused by Low GABA or Serotonin?"
64   Case, "IBS and Serotonin."

PHYSICAL BALANCE. Be careful with your supplements, as some of them can cause what's called serotonin syndrome, the presence of too much serotonin in the gut. If you know that your serotonin is seriously imbalanced, consider working with a professional to select supplements and set up the right diet. You might need prescribed medications too. In general, however, you can focus on eating a healthy diet, getting enough exercise, walking in natural sunlight, going for massages, and balancing your mood with play versus athletic time.

SUBTLE BALANCE. There are a couple of significant activities I'd recommend. These are as follows.

- Go for gratitude. To get to healthy levels of dopamine and serotonin, splurge on gratitude. Science shows that when we express and receive gratitude, our brain releases those two molecules. We become freed of unhealthy emotions and subsequently experience more happiness.[65] So get grateful three times a day. Really.

- Stop. Breathe. Conduct Sports Spirit. Then be thankful. Express thankfulness as often as you can to others, and if you can, ask others to share what makes them grateful for you.

- Balance the second and seventh chakras. These chakras are the subtle energy baselines for serotonin production. Twice a day, conduct Sports Spirit, request the streams, and put one hand on the top of your head (seventh chakra) and the other on your abdomen (second chakra). Request that the streams balance you at all levels inside each chakra, and between them—body, mind, and soul. Breathe deeply and continue with your day.

Adrenaline: The Charge-You-Up Molecule

Adrenaline is one of several molecules or hormones produced by the adrenals.

Adrenaline is more formally called epinephrine, and it feeds your stress reactions. When you are stimulated, such as on game day, epinephrine creates a surge of energy and all the bodily reactions that follow.

---

65   Chowdhury, "The Neuroscience of Gratitude."

This is exactly what you need in order to get up and go. Adrenaline makes your heart pump and your muscles move, and is the key to athletic performance. I also believe that a lot of the negative p's associated with sports involve overstimulation of adrenaline and the inability to get out of our fight-or-flight syndrome.

Think about it.

We can become paralyzed when we just can't manufacture that adrenaline again.

We might procrastinate if we burned through so much adrenaline that our adrenals say, "We're still on vacation."

We might become perfectionist if we've trained ourselves to try only if we think we can do it "just so."

If you've overcharged your adrenals with too many demands, it can take months to recover. Here are ways to do so.

PHYSICAL BALANCE. Create a healthy diet, and work with a naturopath to consider the best supplements. I recommend using one of the many apps for athletes that track micro and macro nutrients and all your dietary needs. Refer back to chapter 7 and the many food suggestions there. Make sure you create downtime and spend more time outdoors. Add Epsom salts to your bathtub water; they contain magnesium, which is a tonic for adrenal fatigue. There are also magnesium lotions for the body.

SUBTLE BALANCE. I'm going to give you something easy and fun to do that is actually bolstered by scientific research: Get thee to a forest or the sea—at the least, to a tree or a babbling brook.

Trees and moving water produce negative rather than positive ions, and the former are better for you than the latter. Positive ions are atoms that have lost one or more electrons and are therefore missing some. Negative ions have gained at least one additional electron. In general, negative ions support our physical and mental well-being, as I'll explain a bit more in a paragraph or so.

Most of us—especially city dwellers—are around too many atmospheric positive ions, which can drain our energy and leave us emotionally depleted and negative. Negative ions are naturally produced by trees and moving water and other natural sites, and even objects like Himalayan salt lamps. In Japan, there is a new term to describe the activity of visiting a forest for its physical and mental benefits. It's called *shinrin-yoku,* or "forest bathing," and studies show that spending time forest bathing is good for the immune system, lowers blood pressure, increases our natural energy, decreases anxiety, depession, and anger, and brings about a state of relaxation.[66]

As I've shared, these "vitamins in the air" are also available from moving water—even the stuff that pours out of your shower! So shower at least once a day. In fact, a study at Columbia University suggests that the positive ions from flowing water might even relieve chronic depression as well as antidepressants do.[67]

I suggest that while you're forest bathing, walking near the water, or standing in your shower, you focus on your first chakra. Ask for the streams to enter and relieve your adrenals. After the calm can come your performance, or at least a little joy.

Vibrational Remedies for the Mind and Emotions: Essential Oils

As you've been learning in this book, there are many ways to employ essential oils. They are excellent for alleviating emotional and mental challenges, supporting forward movement, and bolstering your self-esteem.

I covered how to use essential oils in chapter 4. In addition to the ideas provided there, I suggest that you keep a bottle or two of essential oils in your car or living space. I know many an athlete who takes a whiff once in a while before going into or leaving a challenging situation.

To encourage the use of oils, I'll next outline my recommendations for which oil to use to support the natural conclusion of each of the five feelings, and which to employ to support the increase of specific molecules of joy. It's important to run the use of a specific essential oil by a professional if you are on pharmaceutical medications or dealing with a major medical or emotional life issue, as some oils can be harmful or dangerous if used along with specific meds.

Essential Oils for Specific Feelings

These oils are recommended based on the emotional issue you're working with. Why not use one or many of the suggested oils when conducting all the healing-feeling exercises in this book?

---

66   Li, *Forest Bathing*, 64.
67   Mann, "Negative Ions Create Positive Vibes."

Anger. While using anger remedies, remind yourself to focus on creating boundaries or take a whiff when setting them up. Great oils include bergamot, orange, rose, and ylang-ylang.

Fear and anxiety. You are working on becoming safer, internally and externally. Try the following essences to reduce your tension: bergamot, clary sage, frankincense, lavender, mandarin, and sandalwood.

Disgust. You want to embrace natural feelings of disgust, which indicate that something or someone is bad for you, even while you're releasing shame, a perversion of disgust that leaves you feeling bad about yourself or someone else. Anyone or anything that promotes the sense of being unworthy is a distortion of shame. It's also helpful to forgive yourself and others for failing to have obeyed your own sense of disgust in the past. Support healthy disgust and release the judgments that cause shame with these oils: bergamot, spruce, juniper berry, thyme, citronella, and peppermint.

Happiness. We want more of this! I'll give you a few general oils and more ideas related to specific molecules of joy in the next section: bergamot, frankincense, geranium, lemon, orange, and ylang-ylang.

Sadness. You are allowing yourself to feel into times you've felt unlovable and finding a place in your life for the sport you love. Beneficial oils include bergamot, frankincense, grapefruit, lemon, neroli, and palo santo.

Add-On Tip for Feeling-Based Oils

Did you notice? Bergamot showed up in every one of the previous categories. If you only have the time or money—or nose—for a single fragrance, go with bergamot.

Essential Oils for the Seven Molecules of Joy

When you're focusing on a specific molecule of joy, essential oils provide a fantastic bonus. The sense of smell used to be considered 10,000 times more impactful than any other sense.[68] Research has added an impressive figure to this one. It seems that we can distinguish at least one trillion different odors from each other.[69] That means that an aroma can basically hack into your physical system and change the programs within it. When combining physical and subtle activities with a smell, you bolster the effectiveness of your actions. Basically, you

---

68 Smith, "How Essential Oils Can Boost Your Mood."
69 Zaraska, "The Sense of Smell in Humans."

are using the specific frequencies of an essence to support the positive frequencies of a certain molecule of joy and reduce the negative frequencies causing an "off" neurotransmitter.

The following suggestions will support work with all of the seven joy molecules. Once again—yes, I've said this before—if you are taking a medication, ask a professional about the efficacy and safety of these different oils.

The data provided here is based on a great deal of scientific research I've done; however, I encourage you to do your own if you are really interested in selecting a specific oil for yourself.

Endocannabinoids. Increasing your bliss? Try these oils: black pepper, hemp, clove, and ylang-ylang. Also useful are atlas cedarwood, mastic, chir pine, clary sage, and wormwood.

Dopamine. Looking for your reward molecule? Lavender is terrific, as is oregano, thyme, rosemary, and lemon. You can also go for eucalyptus, globulus, Roman chamomile, and orange.

Oxytocin. Increase that bonding with oils that decrease loneliness, such as bergamot, clary sage, frankincense, and rose. Patchouli will help you fill in the feeling of emptiness.

Endorphins. Get on top of (or under) pain with lavender, rosemary, orange, grapefruit, ylang-ylang, and frankincense. You know what else works? Vanilla, a great anxiety reducer with calming properties.

GABA. Goodbye anxiety with versatile lavender, as well as Roman chamomile. Also try clary sage, rosemary, rose, coriander, fennel, wild orange, lemongrass, and bergamot.

Serotonin. Let's move that confidence up a notch with bergamot, grapefruit, jasmine, and orange. Decrease your insecurities with cedarwood and sandalwood. Lots of good research supports trying bitter orange, rose, and ylang-ylang, as well as lavender, which has a cool constituent called linalool that helps regulate serotonin activity.

Adrenaline. Get charged up when it's time with black pepper, grapefruit, and peppermint. Are you burned out? Go for bergamot, rosemary, black pepper, cypress, and patchouli. In fear? Try bergamot, cedarwood, clary sage, grapefruit, Roman chamomile, vetiver, frankincense, ylang-ylang, neroli, sweet orange, geranium, and rose. Resistant to life changes? Go for wild orange. Need to focus? A little rosemary is called for. Need to push yourself into a necessary (but detested) task? Clementine or peppermint will help! If grief is blocking you from important activities, try cypress, neroli, rose, and sandalwood.

All athletes hit the skids. Maybe you've been there many times or are there right now. When it happens, your mental and emotional condition can suffer. Don't suffer in silence or think you are doomed. Reach out to trusted companions and also employ the subtle energy exercises in this chapter to rebalance yourself. Heal your emotions, learn how to center, get rid of others' energies, employ essential oils, and activate those molecules of joy! And remain hopeful. Life is full of losses and gains; why wouldn't sports be the same?

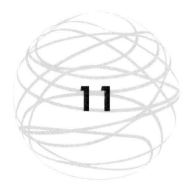

11

Special Chapter for Coaches

It's not whether you get knocked down;
it's whether you get back up.

—Vince Lombardi, former Green Bay Packers coach

For a few months, I felt guided to assist a young teenager in his life. I'll call him Xiao Chen. He was injured playing soccer so often that I got to know the nighttime emergency room doctor. So did Xiao Chen—in fact, it seemed that he liked chatting with the doctor so much that I often wondered if Xiao Chen sometimes manufactured his mini crises just so he could visit.

One time as I watched the doctor bandage a sprained ankle, I asked him how many sports injuries he saw per evening.

"Oh, kids come in here quite often," he said. Then he added, "But you know, my job isn't only to patch up their bodies. It's to show them that they are more than their sport."

The physician was a wise man and a great coach. I hope he's still bandaging kids' souls because that is the essential job of a sports coach.

As a mom in the bleachers, I'm all too aware of the hefty responsibilities associated with being a coach. I'd say pretty much every parent, guardian, or involved grandparent can say the same. Add to this group paid and volunteer coaches, umps, referees, and other game day officiants, and the long list of medical, therapeutic, and training staff involved in athletics, and there is no stopping the list.

Then there is the athlete, who has to become their own coach.

No matter the coaching position you occupy, formal or informal, energy work can help. It can lighten and brighten the burden and add the flavor of fun. And it will help you remain calm, no matter the ups and downs.

In this chapter I'll be speaking to both the external coach and the athlete who is coaching themselves. We'll address intuitive style, and I'll show you how to adapt that to figure out your own coaching style. Then I'll give you tips for assisting both self and other through that style.

I'll also share the importance of boundaries. If you're an external coach, do you really want to be the "midnight coach" reached at any time of day or night? And if you're the self-instructing athlete, come on—you need a little time off.

I'll also speak to certain issues. I can't tell you how many fathers consistently insist that their high school/college/minor league athlete children will never reach their dreams, all because the father never did. Or how many athletes decide to quit a sport—or stay in one— because of the words and actions of a coaching parent or a key authority figure.

A special section in this chapter will assist the external coach of youth with the vital needs of the young athlete, and another will help with the "inner youth" who can be found in both the external coach and the self-coaching athlete. Within each of us are wounded and healthy aspects of ourselves; maybe it's time to heal the first and activate the second.

In the end, so many aspects of sports come down to coaching, which is a role we play. It's such an essential role, the unlocking of an athlete's true potential. That process certainly relates to an athlete's sport and even more importantly to their whole life.

Personality-Plus: Coaching Is a Matter of Style

You've been getting acquainted with your intuition, which we first discussed in chapter 4 in the section called "Intuitive Tools." Remember that I introduced you to four main styles of intuition? Well, the same four styles pertain to both coaching and learning styles.

That's right. We all tend to use one of the four styles more than the others when it comes to becoming educated on a subject, sports included, as well as to informing others. The style you gravitate toward intuitively will be the same one you most naturally use when coaching someone else or serving as your own coach.

To quickly refresh your mind, and also to give you the opportunity to double-check your strongest style, read through the following descriptions. Then consider the one you're most attracted to as your main intuitive style, which will also be your teaching or learning style. You'll be keeping your strongest suit in mind during the rest of this section, while putting your style to work.

Physical Intuitive Coaching Style

You mainly relate to the world through your body or feelings. Yup, you're a doer and an emoter. You seek to accomplish through action, and you seldom sit around. You're also able to assess what is occurring in others' physical or emotional selves through sensations or feelings in your own. Besides staying active, you probably love the great outdoors, or at least you prefer it to being cramped up in a small space and unable to break free to do your own thing.

Spiritual Intuitive Coaching Style

You're all about awareness and consciousness. You're only going to attune to situations and people, or pay attention to what's up, if your value system gives the go-ahead. Prophetic by nature, you love achieving samadhi, that state of oneness with your Higher Power. It can be hard to justify your knowledge of what to do or not do, as you're actually both sensory and philosophical, but if you follow your flow, everything works out.

Verbal Intuitive Coaching Style

It's all about the auditory world. Words, sounds, songs ... you understand through the verbal process, whether that involves what you hear with your physical ears or through your clairaudience, the act of psychically hearing. Even if you don't hear anything, you'll know what's up through the vibrations that move through your body.

Visual Intuitive Coaching Style

You best relate to information and the world in general through visual means. What grabs you are the images you spy with your eyes or those that pop onto your inner mind screen. That "third eye" or clairvoyance sense is the one you trust, especially when you apply it to evaluating appearances and aesthetics.

That's the quick recap. Now for the meat of this section.

Coaches naturally instruct others using their personal intuitive style, expanded to encompass all of reality. That's right. If your coaching style is that of a physical intuitive, you'll be busily sensing what is happening in your athlete's body. You'll sense when they're off, how to best engineer a move, or how much more they can push themselves. If you're an athlete, you'll configure these tendencies to evaluate yourself and become your own coach.

How different things are if you are verbally inclined! Your assessment of an athlete will be based on what they say or maybe on data you've collected through reading. If you're a verbally inclined athlete, you'll need to hear yourself think, get auditory insight from others, or maybe listen to music while working out so you can sense your muscles.

Now I'm going to provide specific coaching tips for the external coach as well as for the self-aware athlete, all based on style. I'll cover your strengths and possible weaknesses, how to zero in on your style, and how to be in integrity with that style. You'll see what I mean.

Physical Coaching Style

Okay, mover and shaker. What's with your style?

FOR THE COACH. You'll naturally assess an athlete based on their physical movements and their obvious body-based skills. You'll be aware of how they move physical and subtle energies and where they flow or get stuck in the body. Simplistically, you'll know what's happening in your athlete's body because you'll sense it in your own. Therefore you'll be great at breaking down mechanics, establishing the right protocol for workouts, and sniffing out emotional blocks. Since you can also intuit another's mental motivations, you'll excel at figuring out how to encourage your athlete. You'll also be terrific at assisting the physical side of your athlete, whether that's with bodywork, doctoring, addressing mechanics, or simply by sharing recommended actions or ways to approach emotions differently.

Can I stretch you? Assist that athlete with differentiating between their own and others' physical and emotional issues. Help them distinguish between healthy and unhealthy motivational drives. It's great if they desire to become the best athlete they can be but not so great if they just want to beat everyone else regardless of ethics. Try your hand at assisting an athlete with clearing negative forces while also accessing and directing the subtle elements, which are quite body-based. You can also work effectively with various natural remedies and even direct your athlete to more powerfully interact with the environment.

Your most obvious weakness will be relating to a non-kinesthetic athlete. You might say "Move your elbow this way" while they just stare at you. Perhaps they are visual, and sensory-based data is a nonstarter. Also, you can confuse your own physical and emotional issues with those of your athlete. Are you sure that your athlete actually has knee pain or is that twinge your own? Motivations can get mixed up too. Imagine your athlete wants to quit or change sports. You might say no if you've fused your own drive with those of your athlete's.

FOR THE ATHLETE. Your ability to assess difficulties and fix them is all about being kinesthetic. That's right. You are body-based, as well as quite sensitive to emotions and the influences of mental motivation.

Want to figure out what's off with a sports concern? Focus on your body and your feelings, and trust your internal conclusions. First, however, make sure you clear out others' energies. You are susceptible to picking up the bodily sensations, feelings, and thoughts of other people, so use the streams to get rid of energies not your own, and then sift and weigh. If you have to make a decision about a person or an activity, listen to your gut—or rather, feel into it. A twisted or sick feeling in your body is a no, while a clear or excited sensation is a yes.

If you really want to care for yourself, make sure you use bodywork, seek out nutritional support, and get lots of sleep. Of all the types, if your body falters, so will your performance.

If you want to make a correction or go in a new direction, you'll have to keep at it. Try something out physically and then see what works. Make bodily corrections. Evaluate for emotional blocks. Be aware of why you want to create a change. Once you land on a desire, anchor it in with techniques like the chain-lock, first clearing out any negative forces. Also, use those subtle elements when you want to fill in an empty hole or get a burst of power. Plant a Vivaxis. Look for signs in answer to your questions coming from the natural world and from what happens around you.

You'll struggle to make appraisals or to implement changes innovatively if you get stuck in your head or in words or if your teachers are visual. You're going to have to feel your way through just about everything. In general, if something feels right for you, it is right for you.

Spiritual Coaching Style

You're the high-minded spirit of the coaching universe. What does that look like?

FOR THE COACH. You believe in your higher knowing. In whatever way you label your Higher Power, that is your source of guidance. It is imperative to trust your conscious awareness, which shows up as a knowing in your being. When seeking guidance for an athlete, tune in through prayer, meditation, or contemplation, and practice how to quickly gain insights.

It probably goes without saying that spiritual intuition can be a difficult coaching style. How do you prove what you know? Compensate for the lack of conclusive evidence by packaging your insights in practical directives. Start statements in these ways: "This is my sense" or "In my awareness, I'd say this is going on." Also ask an athlete to respond to questions by encouraging reflection, like, "What do you do with that discovery?" or "How might you put that idea to work?"

FOR THE ATHLETE. You attune to your sports activities through higher awareness. Sometimes you'll get a sudden knowing or you'll feel like your Higher Power is making something clear to you. If you try to prove the validity of your awareness, however, you'll run into problems—so don't. Simply follow that greater awareness and the sense of destiny that unfolds within and around you. Also consider utilizing prayer, meditation, or contemplation, in the moment or on a regular basis, to receive guidance. Practice the concept of worship (regardless of your religion or belief system) to feel gratitude for what works—and in advance of wanting to receive a sense of direction.

Many self-coaching spiritual athletes receive insights in dreams. These could be night- or daydreams. You can also adapt the dream state to in-the-moment activities. In other words, get good at entering samadhi. Say you're trying to adjust your mechanics. Attempt an alteration and then stop. Be still, if possible. Attune to spiritual guidance and make slight physical adjustments until you're in the flow. Now you have it.

Verbal Coaching Style

Verbose, you might not be—or you might be! No matter how often you verbalize aloud, your style means the following.

FOR THE COACH. You'll know how to support or train your athlete by listening to what they are saying. Focus on the broad strokes but also the minutiae of their speech and language. How do they describe their experience? What's affecting them? You'll examine their specific words and overall meaning simultaneously. And if you're open to it, access a spiritual guide, either your own or the athlete's! It's in your nature to do so.

You can already guess how you'll be supporting an athlete: with words. You'll explain what's needed to the nth degree. Expand. Consider using sounds or noises, like a big *hurrah* when they do something perfect. Play music or certain songs to convey a meaningful message or bolster an athlete's mood. If your athlete is open to your style, assign books, downloads, and even poetry and quotes. Know that you'll excel at hearing an athlete's feelings and desires by analyzing the nuances of what they say and don't say, as well as their tone.

As an aside, consider evaluating an athlete's performance by listening to sports-based sounds, like the sound of the ball on the bat or the clap of cleats on the earth. That snap-crack of the bat not loud enough? Perhaps the batter needs to alter their grip. The cleats are sucking? Maybe your athlete needs to skim the surface more and not land so hard. Sounds give cues and clues to a coach like you.

FOR THE ATHLETE. It's all about sound. You'll best take and give yourself direction if it's verbal in nature. That can include words and statements but also so much more.

What if the ball sounds "off" when you kick it? Adjust. Your hand slap sounds strange on the gymnastics bar? Adjust. You try on a pair of hiking shoes that clump just right? They're the ones to buy! Besides assessing your sports activities via sounds, your training is best done via downloads, reading material, and yes—how you or your guides talk inside your head. Learn how to understand your inner thoughts and how to transform any negatives into positives. Go a step further: set up a litany of affirmations that you run on a loop whenever needed.

Also use your physical voice. Explain what is misaligned out loud and then tell yourself how to make changes. Give yourself lots of pep talks and verbal awards. When something goes right, go lion and roar a huge *yeah*!

Speak your needs to others and heed the guidance provided.

Visual Coaching Style

Put on your performance spectacles and take a look.

FOR THE COACH. You're all about visual input. On the surface, you'll assess an athlete based on appearance. That will clue you in to their needs, to reveal their emotional state; their movements, the key to mechanics; and even the color of an injured area, which will inform best treatment. You'll also offer opinions and advice with visual language, like "I can see what's happening" or "See if you can do this." And you will use visual means to communicate with an athlete, such as by recording videos or otherwise using images and pictures.

Rely on your clairvoyance. Request psychic images. Pay attention to dreams relating to your athlete. As I've suggested many times in this book, psychic messages can come in through the everyday too, so watch for visual signs and symbols in your surroundings. How about employing your imagination? Think about what an athlete wants to accomplish and then let the movie play out in your head and guide you into an idea.

Be careful that you don't assess an athlete on visual elements alone. The appearance-oriented coach might write off an athlete or their mechanics or needs based on surface aesthetics. Is your athlete arriving at practice or an office visit in less-than-savory attire? Put aside visual judgments and go forward until you can determine whether or not the clothing choice is an important factor regarding their performance.

FOR THE ATHLETE. Your decision-making key is visual. Depending on your sport, your optimum workouts are done in front of a mirror, and assessments should involve self- or other-made videos. You'll also thrive by comparing the visuals of your mechanics to those of the experts. And it goes without saying that the pictorial athlete pays a lot of attention to clothing, hair, and other aesthetics. In fact, you'll perform better when working out or engaging in some other athletic activity if you're in a neat and clean environment.

Yes, your inclination gives you permission to buy the latest hot gear in all the coolest colors.

If you're working on new mechanics, try color. Imagine your kinetic segments as different colors, each of which must blend into the others. Remember the kinematics discussion in chapter 6 about familiarizing yourself with geometric shapes? That exercise would work for you! If you're creating a sports plan, write down what you need to do and color code the list, using certain colors for differing activities.

Improve your clairvoyance too. Make sure you're open to receiving psychic inspiration and visions, whether through your physical or inner eyes. Then practice. If you want to succeed at a certain action, picture the accomplishment in your head before you carry it out. Keep going until the image matches the activity. If you ask for signs, input, and insights through your third eye, you'll be constantly shown the way. Just don't judge every book by its cover, including yourself and others.

Coaching Is About Adapting

Chances are that no matter what type of coach you are, you'll have to adapt to someone else's style. There are two sides to that.

- If you're a coach, you'll get your point across better if you customize your insights to your athlete.
- If you're an athlete, you'll be more apt to get what you need if you transform your communication to match your coach's style.

How do you shift styles when you need to?

First, get a sense of the style that matches your athlete or coach. Read through the descriptions of the four types offered at the beginning of our last section with a specific person in mind. Following are a few other clues.

Assessing Someone Else's Style

If you have to figure out someone else's style, these tip-offs will assist you.

Physical Style Tip-Offs

- ▶ Constantly moving, fidgeting, and busy

- ▶ Clearly revealing emotional affect or moods on their face

- ▶ Making use of kinesthetic words and descriptions, as well as verbs like feel, act, do, sense, and desire

- ▶ Bored when asked to sit or listen too long

- ▶ Often displaying emotions and feelings

- ▶ When they do speak, making accurate and insightful comments

- ▶ Glancing only quickly at visual tools or objects

- ▶ Interacting with what is around them, such as through touching or smelling

- ▶ Loving interaction with nature and sensitive to the environment

- ▶ Using words like feels, smells like, did, do, threw, fell, and others that are kinesthetic

- ▶ When you're providing instruction, physically mimicking your ideas

Spiritual Style Tip-Offs

- ▶ Give off an aura of deep self- and otherworldly awareness

- ▶ Emanate a sort of indescribable light

- ▶ Speak in terms that are frequently philosophical or higher minded

- ▶ Respond best to higher ideas or ideals

- ▶ Need the big picture to change

- ▶ Are often mystically inclined

- ▶ Use words or phrases like these: comprehends, understands, knows, is aware of, has a sense of, been revealed, after meditating, upon praying, is aligned, and other higher-concept terms

Verbal Style Tip-Offs

- ► Frequently speaks, hums, reads, writes, or performs some other type of verbal interaction
- ► Often takes time to think before they can understand something
- ► Has to talk aloud to get to a decision
- ► Gains the majority of their sporty insights from discussions, books, downloads, and the like
- ► Often trains or performs while connected to books on tape, earbuds, or music pumped into the gym
- ► Responds best if you talk directly to them; then again, also clues in to the sounds and conversations going on around them
- ► Employs words like these: hears, reads, knows, understands, listened to, was told

Visual Style Tip-Offs

- ► Has a thing for their appearance
- ► Is often fussing with their hair, clothing, or sports equipment
- ► Likes to watch their workouts or other sorts of activities in the mirror
- ► Uses pictures or videos to assess themselves
- ► Will mess with your appearance
- ► Has the neatest and most perfectly designed workout gear and bag
- ► Plans the visuals of a situation down to a tee
- ► Uses words like these: sees, spots, spies, observes, looks, and watches—and language with lots of visual descriptions, such as those acknowledging shape, color, and form

Adapting to Someone Else's Style

Okay, it's time to shift your style to convey a message to your athlete or coach! Here we go.

Physical Style Adaptations

- ► Mirror their physical movements
- ► Reveal your feelings or moods facially

- As is appropriate, demonstrate techniques or what you need

- Use hand, arm, and other gestures

- Show—don't tell—what you mean

- When appropriate, pat them on the back or touch them in some other nonsexual way

- Let them copy what you are trying to demonstrate, whether you are instructing or trying to share a problem

- Teach or talk while they are moving; better yet, while they are throwing a ball, walking, or performing the sport

- Interact with the objects around you; use objects to make your point

- If possible, do needed activities outdoors or in nature

- Get a sense of their inner motivation and align with it

- Use active verbs and words like these: do, show, act, shift, feel

Spiritual Style Adaptations

- Be yourself. Really. The spirit-filled can tell if you aren't being genuine.

- Come from your value system and ask for assistance from that place. Literally, you can say, "This is what I value. How can I help you/you help me..."

- Share your higher goals and aspirations, or what you believe these might be for them

- Come from the big picture

- Go for what is ideal

- Be honest about your beliefs (or lack thereof) in a Higher Power, and emphasize philosophical concepts

- Put the task in the context of greater desires

- Use words or phrases like these: understand, comprehend, consciousness, become aware of, been led to know, have the sense of

- Share your mystical insights and dreams and ask for the same from them

Verbal Style Adaptations

- ▸ You can't just demonstrate or show; give verbal instructions
- ▸ State the message aloud or write it down
- ▸ Can't come up with words? Have them listen to a song with lyrics that encapsulate what you're trying to say, or a book, essay, or phrase that does the same.
- ▸ When they speak, repeat the basic message back to them. Ask if you got it right.
- ▸ Let them take notes or dictate as you go
- ▸ Make sure they repeat aloud what they need to do
- ▸ Emphasize instruction by providing reading or listening material
- ▸ If you're an external coach, encourage the athlete to research reading material about key figures they should emulate.
- ▸ Have music playing in the background
- ▸ Ask them to clue in to the sounds of the sport and then give feedback
- ▸ Package messages with verbal words, like these: hear, heard, read, know, understand, listened to, was told

Visual Style Adaptations

- ▸ Comment on their overall appearance
- ▸ If you are giving or requiring insights, show what you mean. Act out instruction in order to make a visual impression.
- ▸ If you're the external coach, take videos of the athlete and encourage them to do the same for themselves. If you're the athlete, do the same and ask for assessment.
- ▸ Pose questions by demonstrating visually
- ▸ Use Facetime, Zoom, or some other visual medium to communicate when not in person
- ▸ Dress as neat and tidy as possible

- ▸ Keep your equipment organized (if you're the athlete, this will give you brownie points with a coach!)
- ▸ It's okay to share insights that come through dreams or are based on visual signs you receive from the environment
- ▸ Use words like these: see, spotted, spied, observed, look, and watch, and language with lots of visual descriptions, acknowledging shape, color, and form

Shifting to your athlete's or coach's style can really make a difference. For example, I once worked with a basketball player whose father was a former athletic star. This dad just couldn't get through to his daughter.

"I show her the drills, and I've given her books to read," he said. "But she just can't catch on. She makes the same mistake over and over again, and I know I can help her. I mean, I know *exactly* what she needs to do."

As you can guess, we don't always use only a single style. This dad was both kinesthetic and verbal, though he edged toward the verbal style. He'd sit at dinner and explain the moves and steps. Then he'd go out to the court in the driveway and demonstrate. But it didn't make sense to his daughter.

She was partially visual, so she could get the hang of a few of the actions by observing, but not enough to make sense of the drills. I discovered that she was spiritually kinesthetic, which is a different bird altogether. So when she and her father were in my office, I asked her dad to paint the big picture for the daughter. What was the purpose of the specific activity he was instructing her in? How would it benefit her overall game? What did it add to her game in the long run?

The daughter's face lit up. "Oh, I get it," she said. And she did. The next time she was on the court, everything fell into place. A center, she had her best game ever the very next time she played.

It doesn't have to be hard to adjust your style to someone else's. Sometimes a small shift makes all the difference.

Setting Boundaries: How Far to Go

Being an external or athlete-driven coach explicitly means you have to set boundaries, for yourself and for an athlete. Think about it in practical terms. If you're a physical therapist, you have to tell a patient to stretch this far, but not farther. If you're a massage therapist, you're going to press just so on a sore muscle and not deeper or you could cause damage. And if you're an athlete, you constantly have to adjust boundaries when self-coaching. For instance, you have to determine how many lifts you can do before you could get hurt.

As a mom in the bleachers, I know how many situations involve setting boundaries for myself. Can I attend every game? How much money can I reasonably spend for my athlete's training? How much can I help, and in what ways? How do I replenish myself? After all, if I don't, I will lose my own energy. I've always been clear on the need to bring in other coaches, given my personal limitations. First off, I'm not sporty, although I was a pretty good dance line cheerleader in high school and I hike a lot. I also wear many coaching hats and have to have enough energy for the most important one: banker.

No matter what, paid or unpaid, coaches have to think through their parameters. My intention in this section isn't to tell you what your boundaries as an external coach need to be. It's to surface the broad areas for you to consider.

Know, too, that boundaries are a moving target. Those you establish today might need to be shifted tomorrow. That's okay. Just be clear in the present.

Following are the topics to consider. I'll cover both physical and subtle concerns.

Finances. How much money are you willing to spend on the athlete or the expenses related to the sport? If you're the athlete, what's your budget and for what type of coaching? If you're a coach practitioner, what's the minimum fee you will charge to assist?

Time, measurable. What is your time commitment for the athlete, and what concerns are you willing to address and not address? When are you available and during what hours? Will you put in extra, according to your external role, and if so, under what conditions? If you're the athlete, how much time will you commit to your own self-coaching, including research and other activities, and for what reasons would you put in more? How much time can you commit to getting coaching externally?

Time, immeasurable. A lot of sports time occurs on the most important field of all: the mind. Establishing mental boundaries takes a lot of work, but really, you can't spend 24/7 on other- or self-coaching. Even Einstein did his best work while napping, his best ideas springing up when he awoke. So think about the brain space you're willing to give your sport or athlete and how to take time off.

The boundaries of your expertise. I've learned it's vital to be clear as an external coach about what you can offer an athlete and what you can't. One of the reasons my youngest son had to move on from his college is that as nice as the coaches were, they simply couldn't assist him when COVID-19 screwed up his mechanics. Actually, most of his trainers and coaches couldn't, so he had to move on to other pastures. But it wasn't like his coaches made that suggestion. Who did?

I did. So did my dear friend Anthony, who is also my business manager and a respected life coach, and basically like Gabe's uncle. Anthony and I did the "stepping" when the obvious coaches couldn't step to the plate. I know it wasn't because they didn't care; rather, they weren't a good fit for his emotional needs.

If you're an athlete, you need to know what each coach can give you, then stay within their boundaries. As the saying goes, you can't get blood out of a stone.

Emotional boundaries. There are so many feelings involved in being a coach. The same applies to athletes in responding to their coaches. Set boundaries. Don't let all the feelings blur into your personal life. For instance, when I'm working with an athlete client, I focus on them only during our one-hour sessions. Then I'm done. Period. If Gabe calls and has a need, I give myself up to a half hour after the discussion to ponder it, then I move on.

Subtle field boundaries. You can't afford to carry your athlete's subtle energies around with you. And if you're an athlete, you don't want to be burdened by your coach's issues. Use the streams as often as needed to clear yourself.

Mystical boundaries. Our intuitive self is often online even when we're not mentally aware of it. If you're a coach and really involved, that is certainly the case. What are you willing to receive and what aren't you? Sometimes spiritual guides wake coaches up in the middle of the night with a message or vision related to the athlete. Are you okay with that? For me, I've established the rule that I'm cool receiving dreams but not sleep disturbances. You don't want to lose your own life energy for someone else's concerns. As an athlete, you might also have a litany of spiritual guides assisting you. What are your parameters for receiving contact from them? In general, it's always okay to say no to something that is being asked of you, or "I'll get back to you later." That makes your yeses all the more meaningful and productive.

Youth Coaching—for All Ages

Assisting youth—athletes under the age of eighteen—is a special job. There are actually two ways to look at this category, and I'll cover both in this section.

The first subsection is devoted to youth coaches—yup, the "external" individuals who help our youth. The second subsection applies to coaches and athletes of all ages. In that category, I'm going to discuss the very real fact that within each of us, no matter how old we are, dwell multiple inner youth. In therapeutic circles, these aspects of self are called "inner children." To be a really good external coach, or to help yourself as an athlete through all your concerns and opportunities, you need to have a good relationship with these inner selves. I'll help you develop that.

Coaches Serving the Youth

One of the main jobs of all external coaches of youngsters is to support them in finding themselves.

Sports is a vital part of this process for so many youngsters. For some kids, sports is their main outlet—and inlet. More than anything, however, a young athlete wants someone to look up to, to know that someone has their back—and probably front and sides, as well. In whatever way you can, let that someone be you.

Every single coach my kids have interacted with has ended up as either a positive, neutral, or negative role model. That dad coach who yelled at all the football-playing kids? I could see the kids wilt, and those with a tendency toward bullying became more like that coach. The orthopedic surgeon who met with one of my kids when he was injured? The doctor's great attitude and interest in not only my son's sport but in his life still sticks with my son.

Above all, it's important to keep the game fun and understand that kids jump around. Chances are that most kids will eventually quit a sport, but that doesn't mean the sport quits them. Whether a kid shifts from being an everyday athlete to an elite one or not, the impressions you make will remain with them. What do you want to imprint them with: Care? Compassion? Fortitude? The ability to move beyond defeat and to enjoy a success? You might be that person who teaches them a quality that is exactly what they'll need later in their life.

I'll never forget watching a young lacrosse player whose mother had just died. When working with this boy, one of the coaches completely ignored that the death had even happened. Whenever he was in charge of the field, that kid shut down. He would stand paralyzed, unable to move. Another coach often talked to the kid about the loss. When that coach was on the field, the kid shone, often looking over his shoulder to see if that coach was watching him.

Kids at different ages require different types of support. From a subtle point of view, I suggest you return to the rendering of the chakra development ages I presented in chapter 4 and customize your coaching to the issues the youngster is working with at that age. I'll give you a few tips, starting with the youngest age at which most kids start a sport.

Third Chakra, Solar Plexus, 2½–4½. Maybe you've seen those little gymnasts executing cartwheels or baby skiers schussing down a hill. I love watching the tiny soccer players who kick the ball all over the place—and fall all over it—on the field in my neighborhood. Key to assisting kids of this age is keeping in mind the personality traits and abilities they are processing and developing, including the following.

Personal power: This is the age at which a youngster decides how much power they have to effect change around them. Let them do what they can, and show them how to do more. Praise their accomplishments, and if something doesn't work out, help them feel good for just trying.

Positional power: Kids this age are also responding to authority figures and figuring out how much authority they themselves can wield. Model accountability. If you make a mistake, own it. Maybe laugh about it! Don't brag; rather, talk about the skills that led to your own achievements, and if a kid does something great, explain why their actions worked out so well. Give kids of this age responsibilities that are aligned with their capabilities, but also help them when they require assistance.

Belief development: That's right. That third chakra is like a cauldron full of thoughts and observations. In it are thrown the overt messages of coaches and others involved in a sport, as well as psychic messages. Be clean with your own thoughts and as positive as possible. Show kids how to turn a negative experience or thought into a positive one. Above all, deal with your own discriminatory or prejudicial attitudes because kids will pick up on them. Calmly explain to kids why people who are different from them are simply different, not better or worse.

Fourth Chakra, Heart, 4½–6½. Isn't this a fun age? Kids are squirrelly and interactive, have zany personalities, and are ready to rock and roll. They are also developing some pretty keen relational skills, as this age is all about love and relationships. Support them as a coach in these ways.

Social skills: Busy little beavers that they are, these kids are evolving their social skills. It might not always be apparent. Introverts are more internal. They might hang out at the edges—until they power-on for their sport—or only talk to one or two other kids. Those extroverts, though, they'll be running around and chatting. Either type of kid deserves your attention and the modeling of sociability. Show them what it means to be polite, lose with grace, win with humility, and care for others.

Communicating needs: How is a youngster supposed to ask for what they need? Often they don't speak aloud, so pay attention to the signs. Maybe they can't lace a shoe. Be on top of that and, without shaming them, show them how. Perhaps they are acting out or are overly quiet. These could actually be signs that something is off at home or somewhere else. Be open to letting these kids talk to you, and if the situation revealed is really extreme, bring in professional assistance.

Dealing with parents: Okay, I get it. You might be a parent and think you're pretty great, but there are always *those* parents. And no matter what other type of coach you are, you'll be interacting with children's parents or guardians. The little athlete will be watching how you do that. The parent who yells at the volunteer coach? Your response will make a huge difference in how that athlete learns how to relate to others in a similar situation. I remember a conversation I had once during a Little League practice. The athlete's dad confessed that he had come solely to evaluate the coach. "Just to see if there is any modeling we have to redo," he shared.

Fifth Chakra, Throat, 6½–8½. At this stage, it's all about communicating. Even if you don't know kids are listening (or talking, singing, reading, thinking, or playing music), they are. So be aware of exactly what these kids are coming to understand internally.

Acceptable ways to communicate: You don't have to swallow all your words or overdo it, but the way you speak, both audibly and subtly, is teaching kids how to speak and communicate. Obviously, swear words they hear will show up in their own language, but so will sarcasm, prejudice, cruelty, and mockery. Watch your tone too. They are listening.

Philosophies: During this stage, kids are cataloging external communications. In fact, they are creating buckets they can decide to draw from or not. What are these buckets labeled? "What to say when you are mad." "How to ask for what you want." "Ways to deal with a pushy person." Evaluate the concepts you use to run your own life and come from the best ideals possible.

Telepathy: Okay, I have to sneak in a little mysticism. Telepathy is the ability to psychically hear what someone else is thinking. Now, it's not like every kid is telepathic, but they are able to read into what you're saying and thinking. If you struggle with a negative attitude, consider owning it and letting the athlete know what you're working through and how—of course, in an age-appropriate way. Be clear about your own ideals and your young athlete will do the same.

Sixth Chakra, Brow, 8½–14. This stage is all about the visual aspect of life, including several very critical issues of development such as the following:

Self-image: During this age, youngsters are consciously and unconsciously taking in external cues, all of which will determine their self-image. What or who is attractive? Popular? What type of person can become a successful athlete and what type can't? Think about the unlimited sources of data that could be instructing your athlete about their potential and lack thereof. How about the young girl whose parents don't want her to be athletic; rather, they want her to become a doctor or a lawyer? She might not even perceive her athletic capabilities very accurately and may quit prematurely. On the other hand, we have the athlete with a parent who insists they need to eventually go pro—even though they'd rather be a veterinarian or a nurse. Every single idea that burrows into a youngster at this age can impact their sportiness and overall life. Because of this, pay special attention to how you can support your athlete in seeing themselves truthfully, not via comparisons.

Comparison issues: Yup, I just mentioned this factor in the last sentence. Well, this age is all about comparing. It's essential that you watch the athlete for signs, depending on appearances, of everything from sinking self-esteem to pridefulness. Overall, kids are assessing their relative attractiveness, but they are also comparing what they own to what others own. At this stage, some kids might even quit a sport because they think their equipment is ugly. Be sensitive to offering reassurances about these issues.

Heroes: Who are your athlete's heroes? You might be one of them—so be one. Also peruse their list of heroes with them. Ask them what they admire about "person X," and if you need to, gently correct perceptions that are off. "Sure, Mr. Z is crazy on the field, but he also does drugs. How about if you become as cool as him without the drugs?" Help your athlete sort right from wrong.

Seventh Chakra, Top of the Head, 14–21. These are incredibly important years. Overall, the purpose of this stage is to initiate a youngster into adulthood. But there are so many more opportunities than that simple sentence covers. Although we technically consider youth to be adults at age 18, we all know better. Because of this, I'm going to make points that will apply to youth all the way up to age 21, the cutoff time period of this chakra.

Key developmental factors include the following:

Grasping importance: During these years, a youngster must be provided one absolutely essential message: *you are important to the world.* In tribal communities youngsters are ushered into the society through initiation rites. They are encouraged to embrace their unique gifts so they can develop and then offer these to the community. How can you help your athlete understand that the world needs them? Begin to count and master their individual abilities. Their unique attributes certainly might include their athleticism but also, oh, so much more.

Making higher connections: I'm not talking about religion here. I'm speaking of spirituality. During these ages, it's imperative that a young person be shown that they are made of the same stuff as the saints, gurus, and their sports heroes, and they can engineer their own paths. If you are a coach for an athlete during these ages, remember that the way you treat them might become how they treat themselves.

Goal setting: What role will athletics play through this stage? Often during this chakra development period, youngsters quit one sport for another or quit sports altogether. That's because they are evolving into their own special person. Support their process, and for those athletes who decide to go a step further, connect with your own Higher Power to consider how to best assist.

Reprocessing: Between 14 and 21, a youngster is working through seventh chakra issues, such as their relationship to a Higher Power and their own higher self. They are also provided with the opportunity to work through issues related to the lower chakras. In other words, every year between 14 and 21, youth are retriggering issues, events, memories, and capabilities from an earlier stage, so while the seventh chakra is predominant in the overall age range, young athletes are also returning to ages when lower chakras were most active. The following outline might help you customize your coaching to where they're at.

- ▸ 14 to 15: First chakra. Passion, safety, security, trust in and health of the body. During this age, youngsters revisit life concerns, from their worthiness to make money to their ability to make something of themselves.

- ▸ 15 to 16: Second chakra. Emotions and creativity take center stage while these youth figure out in what new directions they will go.

- ▸ 16 to 17: Third chakra. Mentality, ideas, and structure. During this age, a youngster assesses and locks in beliefs about self and the world, and also copes with the need to be structured and organized. The keys to career success are often anchored in this stage.

- ▸ 17 to 18: Fourth chakra. Relationships, love, and caring. It's all about the affairs of the heart, not only regarding romance but also in learning how to be with and relate to peers. Role models help the young person determine their next vital steps.

- ▸ 18 to 19: Fifth chakra. Communication and guidance. The young adult is now determining how they explain themselves to the world and what people (or beings) they are going to consider valid.

- ▸ 19 to 20: Sixth chakra. Self-image and life vision. What are my higher goals? What do I want to become? This is the time period when life goals start to materialize.

- ▸ 20 to 21: Seventh chakra. At some level, this young adult is deciding how to form their world and how to set out on the road ahead. Many athletes are now deciding whether and how their sport might fit into their future.

No matter what type of coach you are, I hope this last section impresses upon you how important you are to the evolving athlete.

The Youngster Inside

We all have a medley of inner children inside ourselves. If you've ever participated in therapy or read a self-help book, you've been introduced to that truth. For both the external coach and the coach athlete, it's beneficial to locate and work with two generic inner youngsters as they relate to athletics:

- the wounded youngster
- the accomplished youngster

In regard to athleticism, the wounded youngster, of any age, is the one who has been hurt physically or emotionally in ways related to a sport. This might be the five-year-old who was made fun of on a field for being slow and pudgy; the kid who was picked on in gym class (that was me); the athlete who sat on the bench for any number of years. This self is actually a collection of wounded inner athletes who combine to form a shock bubble (or several shock bubbles) and who can arise at any time.

Athletes who search often come up with many versions and ages of this self. I remember working with a college hockey player who went pro. His concern was that he freaked out whenever the puck was passed to him. He didn't let the freak-out show, however. In fact, he was a top player in the nation. But he remembered playing a game in fifth grade right after his parents told him they were divorcing. He was so sad that he wet his pants the first time the puck was passed to him. He got through that and every other game that day without letting anyone find out. (There is a lot of padding in hockey!) But from that point on, he'd feel a sharp, telltale pang of fear whenever he received the puck. He used the exercise I've provided at the end of this chapter whenever he was on the ice, and the triggering slowly faded.

Coaches, whether they are parental, medical, or sports related, often have their own inner wounded athlete. Many a professional or youth coach remembers that moment when they were done with their sport at some level. I worked with a coach of a baseball club team who hated going to pro games. He had "washed out" in the minor leagues, and although he loved working with youth, he felt so embarrassed by his "failure" that he would rather skip watching his favorite game than go through the loss again.

At the other end of the continuum, the self-directed athletes and coaches also have accomplished athletes inside. I don't care whether you ever played a team sport; somewhere inside is a self who is proud of their athletic achievements. Although I wasn't much of an athlete growing up, and I still have an intense fear of stray balls flying my way, I was great on the cheerleading dance line. I could actually land on the ground in the splits after leaping into the air. Every so often, I get in touch with that cool self and feel that sense of thrill. When I'm on a difficult hike, my current sport, I remind myself that I used to be able to perform that maneuver. Of course I can make it up the side of a mountain, I tell myself. I used to do the splits! In fact, years ago, I biked through Europe. Even then, reminding myself that I could once land in the splits got me up the Alps.

Coaches, too, can draw from their athletic accomplishments. I have a friend who coaches wrestling and was quite well known in the sport before retiring. When he's helping the youngsters, he thinks about how it felt when he went from zero to something. He knows all the ups and downs, and that assists him in bolstering the kids when they are going through a challenging time.

You're never going to fully retire your wounded young athlete, but you can get them to assist you. Neither do you need to release your accomplished young athlete. Work with either or both using this last exercise in this book.

EXERCISE 58: THE YOUNG ATHLETE(S) INSIDE

If you feel the trigger of a wounded youth athlete or want to better activate an accomplished young athlete, follow these steps as they pertain to you.

Conduct Sports Spirit and then ask for whatever streams the guidance knows you will need. Then walk through both or either of these steps.

1: Get in touch with the young wounded inner athlete who lies deep inside and is now trying to get your attention. Focus on how and why they are reaching your conscious self. Are they physically triggering you at certain times? Causing emotional distress in reaction to a specific stimulation? Maybe you're aware that they are constantly there, watching you work out, perform, or coach, wanting to be tended to. Simply request that your intuitive aptitudes be fully activated so you can better perceive this self. Then obtain more details.

Get a sense of their age and the circumstances that caused them injury. What happened? Let that inner self relate to you how that event or treatment has been affecting them, and also what they need to feel understood and heard. Spend time in relationship with that self and then ask guidance what you need to create healing and transformation. Ask for additional streams, but also ask to be shown if there are any practical activities to conduct. Perhaps you must continually speak with this self or provide reassurance about what happened. When you're finished with this step, continue to the next one or release yourself into the day.

2: Connect with the accomplished young athlete. Linking with guidance, request that your intuitive faculties be fully awakened. Then ask to be made aware of the inner accomplished athlete. What age is this self? What sport or sports were they involved in, and in which ways? What circumstances helped them feel so good about themselves, full of pride and self-esteem? How is this self continuing to instruct your current athletic or coaching self, and are there other ways you can bring them forward?

If you also bonded with your wounded youthful self, ask if it would be beneficial to link the accomplished self with the wounded one. What can they provide each other? Let them remain in communication for as long as needed. When you are finished with this undertaking, feel gratitude for the sport you have so loved and return to your life.

There are hundreds of different types of coaches. Athletes, too, can consider themselves their own coach. In this chapter, you learned ways to approach yourself as a coach no matter your role, including how to assess your natural coaching style. Whether you are instinctively styled toward the physical or spiritual, or are verbal or visual, you were given tips to coach self or other. You were also shown how to adapt to someone else's style. And by embracing any wounded or accomplished youth athletes inside you, you gave yourself yet another gift. You let your history support your present.

CONCLUSION

The five s's of sports training are stamina, speed, strength,
skill, and spirit, but the greatest of these is spirit.

—Ken Doherty, Irish professional
snooker player and commentator

How does your sport energize you?

Do you feel an emotional thrill at the thought of getting out there? Passionate about the physical expression involved? Happy to be part of something bigger than yourself? Or maybe what exhilarates you is the thought of coaching—supporting one or more people in meeting their sports goals.

If that sport is a vital extension of your true self or spirit, then consider yourself an athlete. That makes the path of athleticism extraordinarily important to you.

It doesn't matter if you are an everyday or an elite athlete or perhaps fall somewhere on the continuum between those two. Neither does it matter whether you are a super performer or you never stand on your sport's equivalent of a pitching mound—or a victory podium. You know what really counts: that your sport is a journey into yourself. That means you deserve to embrace the concepts in this book and apply the exercises that are right for you to your sport—and your life.

After all, sports are about energy. Energize your sports life, and you will energize the entirety of your life.

Energy is information that moves, and everything is made of it. As you learned in this book, more than 99 percent of the energy that composes your body, and this world, is subtle, or invisible. For decades, the sporty have been able to improve performance, tend to injuries, and bolster their confidence through hundreds of practices, but not so much through energy work. Energy work recognizes that if you make a small shift in the subtle realm, it's possible to produce great transformation in the physical world.

As you've read and worked with the information I've presented in this book, you've acquired an "energy worker" perspective. You've put on those special energy eyeglasses. You've accessed and enjoyed your intuition for problem-solving, for healing purposes, and for connecting with spiritual allies. You've gained insight into digging for the underlying cause of a sports-related issue and used a tool kit of techniques to create solutions. You can now neutralize negative energies while attracting positive ones, compose workouts that work, and build teams for support.

Likewise, you've been supported in improving your mechanics and soothing injuries through subtle mechanisms. As well, you've turned yourself into a coach, for yourself or someone else or both. And you've also made peace with the ever-changing roles that sports might play in your life. As life happens, our interaction with a sport doesn't stay the same. We evolve, and our relationships do too, including our relationship to sports.

One of the most striking reasons to continue incorporating the energy principles and processes in this book into your sports life and your everyday life is that the sports world is finally catching up with the world of energy. I've emphasized the importance of emotional and mental health throughout this book, providing practical and subtle practices for improving both. For over five thousand years, energy work—energy medicine—has professed that we need to treat ourselves as whole beings. Healing practitioners in the mountains of China, the deserts of the Sahara, the jungles of Peru, the savannas of Africa, and the forests of Lapland have always treated a person as a being, not a doing—as someone composed of body, mind, soul, and spirit.

Metaphorically, no matter if we are an everyday or elite athlete—or something in-between—we can all hold high the meaning behind the Olympic torch and the five Olympic rings. We can all serve what they represent, as related to sports.

The flame itself holds high the values of physical fitness, unity, competition, and love of sport. We know without a doubt that physical fitness and psychological and spiritual well-being are interdependent. Unity can be measured externally but must be fundamentally achieved internally. Competition is a worthwhile activity, but only if it continues to invite balance and keeps us loving our sport.

In addition to its famous flame, the Olympic Games employ a symbol of five rings. I believe that these five rings relate to the values and applications of energy medicine even more than the flame does. Ultimately, they symbolize a united world, fitness of the whole self, and care for humanity.

Energy workers have always acknowledged the truth of living beings. Yes, we are divine. We are, and have, a spirit. We are also material. It is only humane to embrace our very human needs and be glad for them.

RECOMMENDED RESOURCES

Books About Chakras

Dale, Cyndi. *Complete Book of Chakra Healing*. Llewellyn Worldwide, 2009.

———. *Llewellyn's Complete Book of Chakras*. Llewellyn Worldwide, 2016.

———. *Llewellyn's Little Book of Chakras*. Llewellyn Worldwide, 2017.

Books About Energy

Dale, Cyndi. *Energetic Boundaries*. Sounds True, 2011.

———. *Energy Healing for Trauma, Stress & Chronic Illness*. Llewellyn Worldwide, 2020.

———. *The Subtle Body: An Encyclopedia of Your Energetic Anatomy*. Sounds True, 2009.

———. *The Subtle Body Coloring Book*. Sounds True, 2017.

———. *The Subtle Body Practice Manual*. Sounds True, 2013.

Gerber, Richard. *Vibrational Medicine*. Bear & Company, 2001.

Jain, Shamini. *Healing Ourselves: Biofield Science and the Future of Health*. Sounds True, 2021.

Oschman, James. *Energy Medicine*. Churchill Livingstone, 2015.

Books About Energy and Beliefs

Lipton, Bruce. *The Biology of Belief*. Hay House, 2016.

Morter, Sue. *The Energy Codes*. Simon & Schuster, 2019.

Nelson, Bradley. *The Emotion Code*. St. Martin's Essentials, 2019.

Books About the Nature of Your Divinity

I recommend the books by Gregg Braden, including the following:

The Divine Matrix. Hay House, 2006.

The God Code. Hay House, 2004.

The Wisdom Codes. Hay House, 2020.

Books About Past Lives and Other Mystical Phenomenon

Howe, Linda. *Healing Through the Akashic Records*. Sounds True, 2016.

Kaehr, Shelley. *Healing Your Ancestors to Heal Your Life*. Llewellyn Worldwide, 2021.

———. *Meet Your Karma*. Llewellyn Worldwide, 2020.

MacLeod, Ainslie. *The Instruction: Living the Life Your Soul Intended*. Sounds True, 2009.

Walden, Kelly Sullivan. *I Had the Strangest Dream … The Dreamer's Dictionary*. Grand Central Publishing, 2006.

Walden, Kelly Sullivan, and Rassouli. *The Hero's Dream Journey Oracle*. Blue Angel, 2019.

Books About Natural and Spiritual Guides

Andrews, Ted. *Animal Speak*. Llewellyn Worldwide, 2002.

Lembo, Margaret Ann. *The Essential Guide to Everyday Angels*. Llewellyn Worldwide, 2020.

Seidelman, Sarah Bamford. *The Book of Beasties*. Sounds True, 2018.

Books About Healing with Sound

Cousto, Hans. *The Cosmic Octave*. LifeRhythms, 2015.

Goldman, Jonathan. *Healing Sounds*. Healing Arts Press, 2002.

Levitin, Daniel. *This Is Your Brain on Music*. Plume/Penguin, 2007.

Books About Mental Fitness for Athletes

Ericsson, Anders. *Peak*. HarperOne, 2017.

Epstein, David. *The Sports Gene*. Portfolio, 2014.

Galloway, W. Timothy. *The Inner Game of Tennis*. Random House, 1997.

Hutchinson, Alex. *Endure*. Custom House, 2021.

Kuhn, Aihan. *Brain Fitness*. YMAA Publication Center, 2017.

Syed, Matthew. *Bounce*. Harper Perennial, 2011.

Books about Vibrational Medicines

All the following books by Margaret Ann Lembo are simple and effective guides to working with various vibrational remedies.

Animal Totems and the Gemstone Kingdom. Llewellyn Worldwide, 2018.

Chakra Awakening: Transform Your Reality Using Crystals, Aromatherapy & the Power of Positive Thought. Llewellyn Worldwide, 2011.

The Essential Guide to Aromatherapy and Vibrational Healing. Llewellyn Worldwide, 2016.

The Essential Guide to Crystals, Minerals and Stones. Llewellyn Worldwide, 2013.

Books about Yoga Recommended for Healing and Sports

I recommend the books by Lauren Walker, including the following:

The Energy Medicine Yoga Prescription. Sounds True, 2017.

The Energy to Heal. Sounds True, 2022.

Books and Organizations About Geometric Shapes and Their Applications

Featuring BioGeometry, a unique approach to color and geometry created by Dr. Ibrahim Karim of Cairo, Egypt: Karim, Ibrahim. *BioGeometry Signatures: Harmonizing the Body's Subtle Energy Exchange with the Environment*. CreateSpace, 2016.

Lawlor, Robert. *Sacred Geometry: Philosophy & Practice*. Thames & Hudson, 1982.

Organizations Related to BioGeometry

BioGeometry: https://www.biogeometry.ca/home

Vesica Institute: Run by Robert Gilbertand featuring the science, products, and classes about BioGeometry: https://vesica.org/

Organizations Recommended for Education and Training in Energy Modalities

Association for Comprehensive Energy Psychology (ACEP). Provides information and training in using Emotional Freedom Therapy: https://www.energypsych.org/

Daniel Benor, MD, website. Books and research about the effectiveness of energy medicine: https://www.danielbenor.com/

Healing Touch Program. Data, education, and training in hands-on energy healing: https://discover.healingtouchprogram.com/htp-home

International Association of Reiki Professionals. Information about and connections to Reiki healing professionals: https://iarp.org/

Recommended Fitness and Athletic Apps

Adidas Runtastic. For runners and outdoor fitness athletes.

Fitocracy. Free, plus add-on workouts for all levels.

Fitquote. Fitness quotes to get you going.

Freeletics. Short body-weight workouts and coaching.

HUDL. Technique analysis for individuals and teams.

JEFIT Workout Planner Gym. Beginning to advanced; much is free.

Map My Fitness. From Under Armour, fitness and nutrition for all levels.

MyFitnessPal. Comprehensive app for fitness and food

NTC+ (Nike Training Club). Sometimes hosted by celebrity athletes for all levels of help.

Pear Personal Fitness. World-class coaches; only free for two weeks.

SleepTime—Azumio. Support in monitoring sleep.

Strava. Social media app to workout with friends.

Recommended Meditation Apps

Breethe. Popular and functional.

Buddhify. Meditation and peacefulness.

Calm. For sleep.

Happy Not Perfect. Feel-good and great for beginners.

Headspace. Simple meditation and sleep.

INSCAPE. Guided meditations.

Insight Timer. Sleep and relaxation.

iBreathe. Deep breathing for stress.

Meditation Studio. Featured teachers.

Sattva. Inspirations, chants, and more.

The Mindfulness App. Become present, beginning through advanced.

Books and Organizations for Sports in General

Bergland, Christopher. *The Athlete's Way: Sweat and the Biology of Bliss.* St. Martin's Press, 2007.

Athlete Ally. Athletic equality across NCAA organizations: https://www.athleteally.org/

Athletes for Hope. Connecting athletes to charities: https://www.athletesforhope.org/

Challenged Athletes Foundation. Meeting needs of challenged athletes: https://www.challengedathletes.org/

USADA. Free nutritional tips for athletes: www.usada.org/athletes/substances/nutrition

Highly Recommended Individuals

I have a handful of individuals I would recommend for any athlete or coach, no matter your level of development or goals. Following is a mix of coaches, bodyworkers, and even podcasters.

Anxiety and Performance Coaching: Amanda Huggins

Amanda lives what she preaches and has helped endless individuals I know with their deeper confusion and anxieties about the world and themselves as a professional anxiety coach, trainer, and teacher. She offers one-on-one coaching and online classes.

Her courses are integrative, featuring a body-mind-soul approach, and she'll meet you exactly where you are at. Courses include Abundance; Relationship Anxiety; and an Introduction to Anxiety Management. Amanda also works specifically with athletes on manifestation, performance visualization, mindset, and inner dialogue training. If you can swing it, I recommend working with her one-on one. Her stuff works.

www.amandahugginscoaching.com/

Bodywork: Debby Stanley

Debby has numerous bodywork specialties and puts them together in a way that is applicable for the professional or everyday athlete, as well as any other physical concern, such as injury prevention and repair, increasing flexibility, posture repair, and so much more.

One major approach included in her medicine kit is structural integration, a holistic system that approaches the body as a tensegrity structure in relation to gravity. It promotes a rebalancing of the musculoskeletal system, given that the body compensates for strains, trauma, aging, injuries, overuse, poor posture, and more over time. (And think of what the athlete is doing to their body!) I recommend the structural integration in general, and Debby specifically.

Located in Charlotte, NC, Debby is trained in structural integration and also yoga postures, Thai yoga massage, Jin Shin Do (mind-body acupressure), NeuroKinetic Therapy (NKT), Selective Functional Movement Assessment (SFMA), Active Release Techniques (ART), and the Anatomy Trains Structural Integration (ATSI). This arsenal of tools and techniques helps her view the body and its movement with a keen eye for treating the myofascial tissue so she can customize a treatment strategy.

www.debbystanley.com; 704-641-7954

Performance and Life Coaching: Brandon Thielk

Brandon works with clients to shift perceptions and balance the nervous system to neutralize past experiences that have created doubt, fear, and limitation. He uses these experiences to extract valuable life lessons and teach practical skills that empower his clients to step more fully into themselves and align with an enhanced vision for the future.

He utilizes somatic techniques and self-awareness practices to unpack, process, and educate clients, facilitating accelerated growth and learning. Brandon's clients are high-performance focused, including amateur and professional athletes, business professionals, and growth-minded individuals. Brandon specializes in mindset, emotional balance, leadership development, self-awareness training, emotional intelligence, high-performance, conflict resolution, and relationships.

www.evolvedathlete.co

Brandon@evolvedathlete.co

Instagram: @evolvedathlete

High-Performance Pitching Coaching: Ryan Morris, the Baseball Mechanic

Ryan is a former professional MLB pitcher and a highly in-demand pitching coach. He uses his unique background and skill set, including his capabilities as a biomechanics specialist, to develop athletes to their most powerful level. His coaching facilities can assist high school, college, and professional pitchers. His performance coaching draws on his experience with the psychology and impact of energy on athletes. He is located in North Carolina and sometimes conducts immersion experiences for athletes.

https://www.linkedin.com/in/ryan-morris-29663937/

4loveofthegame2@gmail.com

Athletic Coaching and Energy Healing: Cyndi Dale

YES! I love to help athletes! I have a workout/baseball pitching studio in my back yard for clients who fly in to work with me. I also work virtually with athletes and coaches. If you arrive in person, I promise that my dogs (Honey and Lucky) are great ball fetchers, too.

I'm an energy healer, so that's what I concentrate on. I assist clients with examining and clearing ancestral, past-life, and this-life blocks so they can achieve their athletic potential. I'll assist you too with releasing others' energies and showing up as your most empowered self in all areas of life—during your athletic endeavors and long after. Energetics can often assist with injury recovery and that all-important task of making decisions about your athletic present and future as you go.

Cyndidale.com

Life and Performance Coaching: Anthony J. W. Benson

Success is often a matter of healing, growing, and evolving. Anthony works with everyday to pro athletes seeking to improve their performance and sense of self and those ready to move into their next chapter of life.

He blends creative and inner-soul work with practical inspiration through short- and longer-term consulting. His supportive coaching style and beneficial programs meet any athlete where they are—and help move them into a successful future of progressive personal achievement.

https://anthonyjwbenson.com/services/#coaching

Podcast—Your Superior Self: Trey Downes

Real conversations and the art of becoming. That's my takeaway on Trey's interviews, with superior consciousness thrown in.

A husband, father, and pursuer of truth, Trey was on the search for happiness. Sports was a stop on the road. Then the universe sprinkled his life with breadcrumbs, whispering that he needed to get the podcast going... and there is so much more on his road.

Trey interviews top visionaries in the fields of psychology, healing, intuition, and consciousness. He will help you self-actualize by making higher concepts real and down to earth, including gratitude, self-development, and connection with the higher consciousness.

www.treydownes.com

Podcast and Blog—Mind Body Peak Performance: Nick Urban

Nick is a man on the move, and he wants to make sure you are the same! His show presents thorough explorations of all aspects of you so you can maximize your performance. Many of his featured interviewees are on the frontier of bioharmonizing and biosynergizing (listen to him for definitions). Basically, his podcast blends ancient concepts and truths with modern and energetic medicine. Nick's all about helping you fire on all cylinders, whether it's on the sports field or in the board room. He goes into topics you might have a hard time pronouncing, but believe me, they are leading edge: biohacking, nootropics, self-coding, hyper-productive flow state, super fantastic molecules, and so much more.

https://mindbodypeak.com/podcast-welcome/
https://outliyr.com/

Cognomovement: Bill McKenna and Liz Larson

Energy work made real through cognomovement therapies. I love the teachings of Bill and Liz, who combine chakra knowledge with high-level energetics to aid people (including athletes) with all issues. Their commitment to assisting people with deep healing has resulted in the presentation of techniques that can often easily and quickly clear old trauma while activating inner powers.

Just to give you a taste of what is possible, you can turn to exercise 48 to follow one of Liz's practices for programming the body to move in a new way.

www.cognomovement.com

BIBLIOGRAPHY

Benor, Daniel J. "Distant Healing." http://www.aquarianblessings.com/a-distant.

Bergland, Christopher. *The Athlete's Way: Sweat and the Biology of Bliss*. New York: St. Martin's Press, 2007.

Bohra, J. S. "Response of Mustard and Chickpea to the Blessings of Guruji." Department of Agronomy, Institute of Agricultural Sciences, Banaras Hindu University, Varanasi (2006).

Braun, Perrin. "Potassium: Don't Sweat It!" Inside Tracker (blog), November 3, 2014. https://blog.insidetracker.com/potassium-dont-sweat-it.

Brogan, Caroline. "The Surprising Depth of Crystal Patterns in Human Bone." Imperial College London, May 4, 2018. https://www.imperial.ac.uk /news/186129/the-surprising-depth-crystal-patterns-human/.

Brooks, Amanda. Run to the Finish (blog). https://www.runtothefinish.com /marathon-quotes-to-inspire-training/.

Brown, Larry. "Famed Throwing Coach Impressed By Tom Brady's 'Beautiful' Mechanics." Larry Brown Sports, 8/26/2021. https://www.msn.com/en-us /sports/nfl/famed-throwing-coach-impressed-by-tom-bradys-beautiful -mechanics/ar-BB18mGhW.

"Can Athletes Drink Too Much Water?" Beth Israel Lahey Hospital. https://www .winchesterhospital.org/health-library/article?id=13802#:~:text=One%20 recommendation%20is%20to%20consume,fluid%20needs%20and%20drink%20 accordingly.

Case, Christine. "IBS and Serotonin: The Brain-Stomach Link." *Healthline*, November 5, 2020. https://www.healthline.com/health/irritable-bowel -syndrome/serotonin-effects.

Chowdhury, Madhuleena Roy. "The Neuroscience of Gratitude and How It Affects Anxiety & Grief." *Positive Psychology*, May 26, 2021. https://positivepsychology .com/neuroscience-of-gratitude/#:~:text=When%20we%20express%20 gratitude%20and,feel%20happy%20from%20the%20inside.

Cohn, Patrick. "Sports Visualization: The Secret Weapon of Athletes." Peak Performance Sports (blog). https://www.peaksports.com/sports-psychology -blog/sports-visualization-athletes/#:~:text=When%20athletes%20visualize%20 or%20imagine,your%20brain%20for%20successful%20outcom.

Coleman, Erin. "What Is the Percent of Daily Calories That an Athlete Should Consume?" *SFGate*, December 27, 2018. https://healthyeating.sfgate.com /percent-daily-calories-athlete-should-consume-10323.html.

Cousens, Gabriel. *Spiritual Nutrition*. Berkeley, CA: North Atlantic Books, 2005.

Cristol, Hope. "What Is Dopamine?" *WebMD*, June 14, 2021. https://www.webmd .com/mental-health/what-is-dopamine#:~:text=Dopamine%20is%20a%20 type%20of,in%20how%20we%20feel%20pleasure.

"The Curious Study of Water Consciousness." *Mitte News Journal*, October 14, 2019. https://mitte.co/2019/10/14/the-curious-study-of-water-consciousness/.

Dale, Cyndi. *Advanced Chakra Healing*. Woodbury, MN: Llewelyn Publications, 2022.

———. *Llewellyn's Complete Book of Chakras*. Woodbury, MN: Llewellyn Publications, 2016.

"Demystifying Acupuncture." *Integrity Women's Health*, April 17, 2017. https://www.myintegritywomenshealth.com/blog-2/2017/4/17 /demystifying-acupuncture-how-exactly-does-acupuncture-work.

Edwards, Makeba. "Axis of Rotation." *Ace Fitness*, February 1, 2017. https://www.acefitness.org/fitness-certifications/ace-answers/exam -preparation-blog/3625/axis-of-rotation/.

Ekeocha, Tracy C. "Effects of Visualization & Guided Imagery in Sports." Thesis, Texas State University, May 2015. https://digital.library.txstate .edu/bitstream/handle/10877/5548/EKEOCHA-THESIS-2015 .pdf?sequence=1#:~:text=Research%20by%20Newmark%20(2012)%20 supports,their%20biological%20outcomes%20and%20performance.

Emoto, Masaru. *The Hidden Messages in Water*. New York: Atria, 2005.

"Endorphins." *Good Therapy*, April 26, 2019. https://www.goodtherapy.org/blog /psychpedia/endorphins#:~:text=Endorphins%20are%20chemicals%20the%20 body,%2C%20fibromyalgia%2C%20and%20other%20issues.

English, Nick. "7 Micronutrients That Are Important for Athletes." *Barbend*,
September 6, 2019. https://barbend.com/micronutrients-for-athletes/.

"Formal Analysis September 11 2001." Global Consciousness Project,
https://noosphere.princeton.edu/911formal.html.

Freeman, Tzvi. "The Kabalah of String Theory," https://www.chabad.org/library
/article_cdo/aid/2136925/jewish/The-Kabalah-of-String-Theory.htm.

Hack, Damon. "When in Pain, PGA Tour Players Turn to Healer." *New York Times*,
August 9, 2007. https://www.nytimes.com/2007/08/09/sports/golf/09golf
.html?_r=0.

Healing Touch Program, Healing Touch Research page. https://www
.healingtouchresearch.com/studies.

Hill, Napoleon. *Think and Grow Rich*. Mankato, MN: Capstone Publishing, 2010.

Hjardar, Kim. "The Truth About Viking Berserkers." *History Extra*, March 19, 2020.
https://www.historyextra.com/period/viking/the-truth-about-viking-berserkers/.

"How to Balance Your Endocannabinoid System." *Cibdol*. https://www.cibdol.com
/cbd-encyclopedia/how-to-balance-your-endocannabinoid-system#nl-subscribe
-popup.

Hunt, Tam. "The Hippies Were Right: It's All About Vibrations, Man!" *Scientific
American*, December 5, 2018. https://blogs.scientificamerican.com
/observations/the-hippies-were-right-its-all-about-vibrations-man/.

International Association of Reiki Professionals. https://blendeventdc.wixsite.com
/skinergy/services2-cgaj.

Johns Hopkins University. "Dark Matter May Be Older Than the Big Bang."
Science Daily, August 7, 2019. https://www.sciencedaily.com
/releases/2019/08/190807190816.htm.

Julson, Erica. "10 Best Ways to Increase Dopamine Levels Naturally." *Healthline*,
May 10, 2018. https://www.healthline.com/nutrition/how-to-increase
-dopamine.

Kettley, Sebastian. "Dark Matter Breakthrough: Mystery Substance 'Exists' and
Explains 90% of the Universe." *Express*, May 2, 2019. https://www.express
.co.uk/news/science/1121154/Dark-matter-space-discovery-dark-matter
-energy-galaxies-universe.

Keyes, Raven. "Reiki in the NFL." *Psychology Today*, Fall 2010. https://www
.psychologytoday.com/files/attachments/48451/reikinfl.pdf.

King, Billie Jean. Twitter, December 28, 2017. https://twitter.com/BillieJeanKing
/status/937665738952921088.

Koberlein, Brian. "How Are Energy and Matter the Same?" *Universe Today*,
November 26, 2014. https://www.universetoday.com/116615/how-are-energy
-and-matter-the-same/.

Laszlo, Ervin. "An Unexplored Domain of Nonlocality." Excerpt from *Quantum
Shift in the Global Brain*. Rochester, VT: Inner Traditions, 2008. http://www
.worlditc.org/f_21_laszlo_scientific_explanation_of_itc.htm.

Leonard, Jayne. "A Guide to EFT Tapping." *Medical News Today*, September 26,
2019. https://www.medicalnewstoday.com/articles/326434#:~:text=A%20
2016%20review%20of%2020,other%20standard%20treatments%20for%20
depression.

Li, Qing. *Forest Bathing*. New York: Penguin Life, 2018.

Lies, Elaine, and Gabriella Tetrault-Farber. "Simone Biles Says Gymnastics Is Not
Everything, 'We Also Have to Focus on Ourselves.'" *Reuters*, July 27, 2021.
https://www.reuters.com/lifestyle/sports/olympics-gymnastics-biles-says
-gymnastics-not-everything-we-also-have-focus-2021-07-27/.

Life Extension. "Magnesium L-Threonate: Brain Benefits." https://www
.lifeextension.com/magazine/2018/6/reverse-clinical-measures-of-brain-aging.

Lower, Matt. "The Separation Is the Preparation." *CoachUp Nation*, January 29,
2014. https://www.coachup.com/nation/articles/the-separation-is-in-the
-preparation-5-steps-to-be-successful-like-seattle-seahawks-quarterback-russell
-wilson.

Mandela, Nelson. Speech at the Laureus Lifetime Achievement Award, Sporting
Club, Monaco, Monte Carlo, May 25, 2000. http://db.nelsonmandela.org
/speeches/pub_view.asp?pg=item&ItemID=NMS1148.

Mann, Denise. "Negative Ions Create Positive Vibes." *WebMD*, May 6, 2002.
https://www.webmd.com/balance/features/negative-ions-create-positive-vibes.

McTaggart, Lynne. *The Intention Experiment*. New York: Atria, 2008.

———. "Evidence." Lynne McTaggart website. https://lynnemctaggart.com /intention-experiments/evidence/.

Michalcyzk, Maggie. "The Best Vitamins for Athletes." *Concordia St. Paul*, April 24, 2020. https://online.csp.edu/blog/best-vitamins-for-athletes/.

Mind Matter News, "Tibetan Monks Can Change Their Metabolism," September 18, 2019. https://mindmatters.ai/2019/09/tibetan-monks-can-change-their -metabolism/.

Osaka, Naomi. "Naomi Osaka: 'It's O.K. Not to Be O.K.'" *Time*, July 8, 2021. https://time.com/6077128/naomi-osaka-essay-tokyo-olympics/.

Payne, Andrew. "Sagittal, Frontal, and Transverse Plane: Movement and Exercises." NASM.org. https://blog.nasm.org/exercise-programming/sagittal-frontal -traverse-planes-explained-with-exercises.

Peace Health. "Vitamin C for Sports & Fitness." https://www.peacehealth.org /medical-topics/id/hn-898006#:~:text=Vitamin%20C%20is%20also%20 important,that%20may%20occur%20from%20exercise.

Perry, Philip. "The Basis of the Universe May Not Be Energy or Matter but Information." *Big Think*, August 27, 2017. https://bigthink.com/philip-perry /the-basis-of-the-universe-may-not-be-energy-or-matter-but-information.

Purdy, Eileen. "Is Your High Functioning Anxiety Caused by Low GABA or Serotonin?" https://www.eileenpurdy.com/blog/2018/1/2/is-your-high -functioning-anxiety-caused-by-low-gaba-or-serotonin.

Quinn, Elizabeth. "Recommended Water Intake for Athletes During Exercise." *Verywellfit*, November 22, 2020. https://www.verywellfit.com/how-much-water -should-you-drink-3120428.

"Randy Johnson." *Biography Mask*, February 23, 2022. https://biographymask .com/randy-johnson/.

Reneau, Annie. "Snowboarding Gold Medalist Chloe Kim Gets Real About Her Mental Health Struggles and Triumphs." *Upworthy*, February 10, 2022. https://www.upworthy.com/chloe-kim-mental-health-olympics?rebelltitem =1#rebelltitem1.

Rivera-Dugenio, Jere. "Scalar-Energy Morphogenetic Field Mechanics." Honolulu: International Quantum University for Integrative Medicine, 2015. http://www

.quantumspanner.com/uploads/7/9/8/8/7988916/scalar_morphogenetic_field
_mechanics_and_nde.pdf.

———. "Scalar Plasma Technology and Water as an Effective Stress Management
Protocol for Healing the Cellular Regenerative System." *Semantic Scholar*, 2017.
https://pdfs.semanticscholar.org/89b6/03211dc1
aed8da4808eff1603195f6a1e24e.pdf.

Roll, Rich. *Finding Ultra*. New York: Harmony Books, 2013.

Russell, Daniel A. "Acoustics and Vibration of Baseball and Softball Bats."
Pennsylvania State University, Winter 2017. https://acousticstoday.org
/wp-content/uploads/2017/12/Acoustics-and-Vibration-of-Baseball-and
-Softball-Bats-Daniel-A.-Russell.pdf.

Sadeghi, Habib, and Shahrzad Sami. "Forgotten Genius: Royal Raymond Rife." *The
L.I.G.H.T*, August 28, 2017. https://behiveofhealing.com/forgotten-genius-royal
-raymond-rife/.

Siegel, Ethan. "Science Uncovers the Origin of the First Light in the Universe."
Forbes, June 30, 2017. https://www.forbes.com/sites/startswithabang
/2017/06/30/science-uncovers-the-origin-of-the-first-light-in-the
-universe/#30128dcc3487.

Sirani, Mike. "Four Easy Steps for Improving Thoracic Rotation." https://www
.mikesirani.com/blog/2017/6/22/4-easy-steps-for-improving-thoracic-rotation.

Skidmore, Ryan. "8 Ways to Sleep Like a Pro Athlete." *Simplifaster*.
https://simplifaster.com/articles/athlete-sleep-habits/.

Smith, Jasmine. "How Essential Oils Can Boost Your Mood." *MindBody*, March 17,
2020. https://explore.mindbodyonline.com/blog/wellness/how-essential-oils
-can-boost-your-mood.

Stojko, Elvis. *Sports Psychology,* December 21, 2010. https://sportpsychquotes
.wordpress.com/tag/energyintensity/.

Sulak, Dustin. "Introduction to the Endocannabinoid System." *NORML*.
https://norml.org/marijuana/library/recent-medical-marijuana-research
/introduction-to-the-endocannabinoid-system/.

Sundermier, Ali. "99.9999999% of Your Body Is Empty Space." *Science Alert*, September 23, 2016. https://www.sciencealert.com/99-9999999-of-your-body-is-empty-space.

Tate, Karl. "Cosmic Wave Background." Space.com, April 3, 2013. https://www.space.com/20330-cosmic-microwave-background-explained-infographic.html.

U.S. Anti-Doping Agency (USADA). "Carbohydrates, the Master Fuel." https://www.usada.org/athletes/substances/nutrition/carbohydrates-the-master-fuel/.

———. "Fat as Fuel—Fat Intake in Athletes." https://www.usada.org/athletes/substances/nutrition/fat/.

———. "Protein's Role as a Team Player." https://www.usada.org/athletes/substances/nutrition/carbohydrates-the-master-fuel/.

University of Adelaide. "Types of Body Movements." https://myuni.adelaide.edu.au/courses/11275/pages/9-dot-5-types-of-body-movements.

"Vagus Nerve Exercises." Anxiety Recovery Centre Victoria. https://www.arcvic.org.au/34-resources/402-vagus-nerve-exercises.

Verma, Prakhar. "Destroy Negativity from Your Mind with This Simple Exercise." Mission.org, November 27, 2017. https://medium.com/the-mission/a-practical-hack-to-combat-negative-thoughts-in-2-minutes-or-less-cc3d1bddb3af.

Vidyapeeth, B. S. Konkan Krishi. "Alphonso Mango—Spongy Tissue." Dapoli University, Department of Agricultural Botany, Dapoli, India, Dr. B.B. Jadhav, Director Report No. ACD/BOT/982/of 2006, June 20, 2006.

Weathers, Jim. http://www.jimshealingenergy.com/index.html.

Wei, Marlynn. "The Healing Power of Sound as Meditation." *Psychology Today*, July 5, 2019. https://www.psychologytoday.com/us/blog/urban-survival/201907/the-healing-power-sound-meditation.

Wilczek, Frank. "Crystals in Time." *Scientific American*, November 2019, 30–35.

Wise, Brandon. "Remembering Muhammad Ali." CBS Boxing, June 4, 2016. https://www.cbssports.com/boxing/news/remembering-muhammad-ali-the-greatest-of-all-time-by-his-10-greatest-quotes/.

Wooden, John. *Life Wisdom: Quotes from John Wooden.* Nashville, TN: Meadow's Edge Group, 2013.

Wylie, Robin. "Olympic Gold May Depend on the Brain's Reward Chemical." *Scientific American*, August 5, 2016. https://www.scientificamerican.com /article/olympic-gold-may-depend-on-the-brain-s-reward-chemical/.

Zahran, Samah Khaled. "Human Bio-field and Psychical Sensitivity." *Journal of Psychology and Psychiatric Studies* 1, no. 1 (July 11, 2019). https://www .innovationinfo.org/articles/JPPS/JPPS-1-107.pdf.

Zaraska, Maria. "The Sense of Smell in Humans is More Powerful Than We Think." *Discover*, October 11, 2017. https://www.discovermagazine.com/mind/the -sense-of-smell-in-humans-is-more-powerful-than-we-think.

Ziegler, Maseena. "Famous Quotes You Definitely Didn't Know Were from Women." *Forbes*, September 1, 2014. https://www.forbes.com/sites /maseenaziegler/2014/09/01/how-we-all-got-it-wrong-women-were -behind-these-7-famously-inspiring-quotes/?sh=f1864f81016f.

Zorn, Eric. "Without Failure, Jordan Would Be a False Idol." *Chicago Tribune,* May 19, 1997. https://www.chicagotribune.com/news/ct-xpm-1997-05-19 -9705190096-story.html.

INDEX

Abduction, 128

Absentee healing, 92, 94

Absolute light, 73, 85, 141, 175, 180, 182, 193, 197, 219

Absolute scalar waves, 72–74, 84

Acceleration, 120

Acupuncture, 3, 57, 220

Addictions, 217

Adding new frequencies, 134

Adduction, 128, 154

Adrenaline, 38, 222, 223, 226

Adrenals, 38, 52, 54, 216, 222–224

Agility, 22, 154

Air element, 134, 199

Ali, Muhammad, 101

Ancestors, 30, 39, 41, 48, 49, 63, 171, 256

Ancestral issues, 53

Anger, 43, 191, 211, 213, 214, 224, 225

Angular motion, 118

Anti-anxiety molecules, 220

Antidepressants, 224

Anxiety, 86, 89, 125, 139, 165, 185, 195, 201, 208, 215, 217, 220, 221, 224–226, 260

Applied kinesiology, 69, 80–82, 150, 151, 184

Athleticism, 16, 37, 38, 48, 61, 125, 153, 174, 248, 250, 253

Atoms, 11, 43, 173, 223

Attachments (subtle), 44, 88, 163, 178

Attention Deficit Hyperactivity Disorder (ADHD), 217

Auric fields/layers, 4, 18, 54, 59, 65, 80, 86, 88, 135, 178

Autonomic nervous system, 39, 197

Axes/axis, 15, 118, 123, 126, 127, 137, 141, 143, 144, 154, 197, 221

Bach Flower Remedies, 157

Badminton, 13, 199

Bandy, 199

Baseball, 1, 11, 25, 26, 29, 30, 60, 77, 101, 103, 106, 112, 128, 146, 147, 169, 176, 194, 199, 205, 207, 209, 219, 250, 261

Basketball, 2, 23, 67, 111, 120, 185, 199, 203, 206, 241

Beliefs, 21, 32, 34, 35, 37, 53, 59, 61, 65, 75, 88, 89, 137, 156, 163, 187, 204, 212, 213, 215, 239, 249, 255

Benchmarks, 24

Benor, Daniel, 92, 258

Benson, Herbert, 116, 261

Bergland, Christopher, 216, 259

Berserkers, 115–117

Bicycling, 199

Big Bang, 73

Biles, Simone, 203, 204, 206

Bioenergetic, 13, 92

Biofield, 172–174, 179, 184, 255

Biomechanically intelligent clothing, 113

Biomechanics, 112, 131, 261

Birkebeiner, 207, 208

Blessing, 16

Bliss molecules, 216

Board of Directors, 152, 192, 201

Body awareness, 172, 174, 175

Body segments, 129

Bonding molecules, 218

Boundaries, 24, 69, 172, 173, 179,
    214, 225, 230, 242, 243, 255

Brady, Tom, 111

Brain, 32, 34, 35, 39, 40, 54, 60, 79, 83,
    116, 165, 166, 185, 186, 197, 205, 212,
    216, 218, 220–222, 243, 256, 257

Brain states, 39, 83, 165, 166

Brain waves, 83, 116, 165, 166

Brain, and sleep, 165, 166, 221

Breathing, 24, 26, 27, 38, 51,
    54, 116, 200, 221, 259

Bumgarner, Madison, 112

Calendar, 155

Calories, 158, 159

Camino de Santiago, 24, 104, 105, 170

Cannabis, 216, 217

Canoeing, 199

Carbohydrates, 158, 160

Cardinal axes, 123, 141

Cardinal planes, 122, 123, 125–127,
    135, 138, 141, 154, 197

Cellular receptors, 216

Center of gravity, 123, 129, 132, 135,
    136, 175, 191, 193, 194, 200

Center point, 15, 118

Central axis, 123, 221

Chain-lock, 69, 78, 80, 155, 166,
    167, 180, 184, 192, 194, 233

Chakra activation ages, 52, 54, 56,
    87, 178, 245, 248, 249

Chakra blocks, 54, 56

Chakra colors, 52, 54, 59

Chakra foods, 157, 158, 163, 164

Chakra sounds, 52, 59, 86

Chakra system, twelve-chakra, 83

Chakra wheels, 78, 80, 86, 135, 136, 139–
    141, 143, 155, 156, 182, 193, 219, 221

Chakras, 4, 17, 18, 21, 24, 38, 52–54,
    56, 57, 59, 65, 73, 75, 78–80, 84–88,
    122, 125, 130, 136–138, 140–143,
    156, 157, 163, 178, 183, 193, 196,
    197, 219, 221, 222, 248, 255

Charges, 40, 43–45, 47, 49, 56, 57,
    63, 88, 128, 165, 176, 178

Chi, 3, 22, 23

Chronic traumatic encephalopathy (CTE), 211

Circles, 82, 118, 144, 244

Clairaudience, 54, 76, 231

Clairvoyance, 54, 231, 235, 236

Classical physics, 112, 113, 115, 116, 144

Coaches, type, 13, 170, 236, 242, 245, 246, 249, 252

Coaching, 23, 25, 49, 59, 65, 113, 114, 155, 156, 170, 171, 208, 230–236, 242, 244, 245, 248, 252, 253, 258, 260–262

Coaching, adapting, 95, 230, 236, 238, 252

Coaching, self, 99, 113, 230, 234, 242

Coaching, styles, 230–236, 238, 241, 252, 262

Coaching, tips, 1, 13, 97, 103, 156, 230, 232, 245, 252

Coaching, youth, 26, 230, 244, 250, 252

Conscious self, 85, 251

Consciousness, 17, 18, 21, 71, 73, 76, 80, 83, 85, 86, 95, 115–118, 128, 134, 135, 142, 175, 199, 217, 231, 239, 262, Cords, 44, 45, 88, 178, 211

Cortisol, 38

Cosmic background radiation, 73

Counterforce, 120

COVID-19, 169, 182, 205, 243

Creation, 118

Crystals, and healing, 257

Crystals, and the body, 95, 96, 174, 175

Crystals, programming, 95, 96, 173, 174

Crystals, space, 173–175

Crystals, space-time, 174

Crystals, subtle energy, 173, 175

Crystals, time, 173–175, 271

Curses, 44, 45, 88, 173, 178

Dancing, 113

Dark matter, 73, 267

Deflection shields, 45, 88, 178

Depression, 89, 140, 208, 215, 217, 220, 221, 224

DeRozan, DeMar, 206

Destiny, 44, 140, 152, 164, 234

Digital forces, 41

Dimensions, 117, 118, 128

Disgust, 213, 214, 225

Doherty, Ken, 253

Dopamine, 216–218, 220, 222, 226

Downward spiral, 4, 9, 25, 36, 204, 213

Dreaming, 192

Dreams, 14, 17, 26, 30, 77, 125, 146, 170, 192, 193, 230, 234, 235, 239, 241, 243

Earth element, 134

Edison, Thomas, 145, 146

Eighth chakra, 76

Einstein, Albert, 117, 242

Elements, 95, 132, 134, 175, 180, 182, 183, 190, 193, 198–200, 202, 232, 233, 235

Elements, for healing, 180–183

Eleventh chakra, 76, 148

Emotional balancing, 22

Emotional forces, 41

Emotional Freedom Technique, 89–91, 150

Emotions, 2, 22, 24, 25, 41, 45, 54,
83, 129, 137, 148, 156, 161, 173,
177, 204, 205, 208, 211–213, 222,
224, 227, 232, 233, 237, 249

Emoto, Masaru, 95, 117

Empathy, 54, 75–77

Empowered consciousness, 18

Endocannabinoids, 216, 226

Endorphins, 219, 220, 226, 266

Energetic anxiety, 139, 215

Energetic boundaries, 24, 172, 173, 255

Energetic constructs/contracts,
40, 41, 44, 48, 138, 173

Energetic depression, 140

Energetics, 2, 5, 7, 9, 19, 21, 23–26, 31,
56, 59, 79, 86, 99, 104, 106, 112, 113,
143, 153, 158, 171, 217, 261, 263

Energy analysis and healing,
69, 86, 150, 204, 210

Energy anatomy, 7, 17, 44, 52

Energy blocks, 30, 32

Energy healing, 255, 258, 261

Energy marker, 9, 45

Energy medicine, 1–3, 30, 254, 255, 257, 258

Energy system, 4, 83

Energy work, 3, 7, 10, 53, 69, 99, 101, 114,
135, 173, 190, 230, 253, 254, 263

Energy, subtle, 2–4, 7, 10, 13, 14, 16–19,
21–26, 31, 34, 37, 41, 43, 44, 51, 52,
57, 59, 68, 69, 72, 76, 92, 95, 96, 102,
112, 113, 116, 117, 129, 131, 132,
136, 141, 143, 144, 153, 157, 158,
161, 162, 167, 171–173, 175–177,
179, 180, 183, 187, 191, 197, 209,
217, 218, 222, 227, 232, 243, 257

Enteric nervous system, 39, 221

Entities, 41, 44, 74, 106, 139–141, 173, 210

Entrance points, 42

Environmental forces, 40

Enzymes, 158, 216

Epigenome, 39, 46, 137

Epinephrine, 222

Equilibrium, 4, 15, 36

Equipment, 13, 157, 171, 173, 238, 241, 247

Essential oils, 96, 186, 205, 224, 225, 227

Ether element, 34

Exit points, 42, 43, 128, 179

Extension, 32, 127, 165, 204, 253

Failure, 4, 17, 46, 60, 63, 102, 106, 107,
109, 153, 191, 203, 204, 207, 213, 250

Fats, 158, 159, 161, 163

Fear, 22, 41, 104, 107, 125, 190, 191, 194,
201, 212–214, 225, 226, 250, 260

Fears, 26, 137, 185, 192, 201

Feeling empathy, 54, 75

Feelings, 18, 23, 24, 33, 34, 37, 39, 40, 42, 51, 57, 60, 71, 75, 89, 137, 163, 164, 166, 177, 182, 190, 191, 201, 204, 206, 211–214, 218, 224, 225, 231, 233, 234, 237, 238, 243

Field (of energy), 128, 172

Fifth chakra, 130, 142, 246, 249

Finances, 242

Fire element, 182, 199

First chakra, 37, 45, 52–54, 56, 59, 75, 87, 130, 137, 142, 157, 158, 162, 178, 197, 224, 249

First Law of Inertia, 118

Five senses, 76, 78

Flexion, 127

Flow, 15, 17, 31, 57, 69, 70, 80, 82, 83, 93, 105, 107, 108, 118, 119, 130–135, 141, 142, 144, 148, 150, 155, 162, 163, 175, 180, 184, 191, 195, 198, 231, 232, 234, 262

Flower essences, 3, 22, 95, 96, 201

Fluidity, 199

Focus, 2, 12–14, 16, 21, 30, 31, 41, 47, 51, 65, 74, 78, 79, 86, 89, 92, 94, 101, 113, 115, 117, 127, 129, 131, 137, 141, 143, 153, 160, 161, 171, 172, 179, 182, 191, 195, 199, 200, 203, 205, 206, 213–215, 219, 222, 224–226, 233, 234, 243, 251

Football (American), 2, 11, 40, 43, 120, 199, 200, 208, 244

Football (Non-American), 111

Force empathy, 76

Forces, 19, 40–44, 47, 49, 54, 63, 76, 80, 88, 108, 120, 121, 123, 128–131, 148, 164, 173, 176, 178–180, 183, 198, 204, 210, 232, 233

Forest bathing, 223, 224

Four-Six Breath Exercise, 26, 51, 195, 221

Fourth chakra, 51, 54, 75, 130, 142, 219, 245, 249

Freedom, 64, 89–91, 127, 150, 185, 258

Frequencies, 4, 11, 20, 21, 26, 43, 52, 59–65, 73, 75, 89, 118, 119, 134, 135, 148–150, 161, 163, 164, 167, 172, 194, 226

Frequencies, negative, 62–64, 148, 194, 226

Frequencies, positive, 62–64, 135, 149, 150, 161, 163, 164, 172, 194, 226

Frequency, 11, 20, 60, 61, 73

Frequency, optimum, 20

Friction, 129

Frontal Axis, 126

Frontal plane, physical, 125

Frontal plane, subtle, 125

Future, 15, 56, 80, 114, 122, 125, 139, 147–152, 154, 155, 157, 161, 163, 184, 221, 249, 255, 260–262

Future-past healing, 139

Gaining spiritual guidance, 69, 78

Game day, 4, 24, 25, 37, 99, 101, 102, 138, 142, 147, 148, 153, 154, 156, 189, 190, 192–194, 198, 200–202, 222, 229

Gameline, 67, 69, 73, 83, 84, 86, 132, 140, 141, 156, 177, 194, 195, 200, 204, 221

Gamma Aminobutyric Acid (GABA), 220

Gamma axis, 128

Gamma Gameline, 67, 69, 73, 83, 84, 86, 132, 140, 141, 156, 177, 194, 195, 200, 204, 221

Gamma, consciousness, 73, 85, 86, 128

Gender, 146, 208

Genes, 54

Geometry, 143, 257

Geometry, and kinematics, 143

Ghosts, 41

God, 33, 35, 68, 71, 115, 134, 256

Golf, 3, 12, 46, 128, 131, 154, 200

Grace, 15, 72, 74, 85, 161, 170, 172, 206, 246

Gratitude, 97, 148, 222, 234, 252, 262

Gravity, 117, 123, 129, 132, 135, 136, 175, 191, 193, 194, 199, 200, 260

Grounding, 85, 125, 132, 133, 137, 193, 199

Gymnastics, 199, 203, 235

Hado, 95

Hands-On Healing, 92–94, 171, 180

Healing, 3, 14, 15, 20, 26, 34, 42, 47, 54, 69, 72–74, 76, 83, 86, 88, 89, 92–94, 139–142, 150, 163, 166, 171, 176, 179–183, 187, 192, 204, 210, 211, 213, 251, 253–258, 261–263

Healing Streams of Grace, 15, 72, 74

Healing Touch Therapy, 92

Higher mind, 32, 34, 35, 85

Higher Power, 3, 33, 35, 56, 68, 71, 74, 231, 233, 234, 239, 248

Higher Spirit, 56, 70, 71, 74, 78–80, 86, 88, 91, 94, 97, 133, 134, 136–138, 143, 148, 152, 156, 161, 163, 166, 179, 181, 219

Hiking, 189, 200, 209, 235

Hill, Napoleon, 152

House, Tom, 111

Hydration, 147, 156, 157, 160, 163, 167

Hypnotherapy, 3

Hyponatremia, 160

Ida, 196, 197

Immune system, 39, 54, 159, 223

Inertia, 118, 119

Inflammation, 48, 159, 176, 181, 187, 216

Information, 2, 5, 7, 10–12, 15, 18, 19, 26, 43, 56, 60, 72, 74, 76, 82, 89, 96, 99, 112, 114, 118, 119, 125, 149, 161, 172, 173, 183, 193, 231, 253, 258

Injuries, 4, 15, 21, 23, 34, 40, 165, 169–171, 176, 180, 181, 186, 211, 216, 229, 253, 254, 260

Injuries, acute, 171, 180

Injuries, care, 3, 4, 23, 169, 171, 172, 176, 186, 187

Injuries, chronic, 171, 180, 181

Injuries, overuse, 171, 176, 186, 187, 260

Injury, prevention, 3, 4, 23, 167, 169, 171–173, 175, 176, 187, 216, 260

Injury, recovery, 3, 4, 23, 36, 48, 169, 171, 172, 176, 183, 186, 187, 261

Inner child/children, 26, 99

Intention, 11, 16, 92, 97, 115, 117, 119, 135, 157, 166, 175, 195, 242

Intuitive, 1, 2, 10, 13, 53, 54, 69, 74, 76–78, 114, 127, 133, 134, 136, 137, 148, 155, 230, 231, 243, 251, 252

Intuitive styles, 69, 76, 77

Intuitive tools, 69, 74, 230

Ions, 223, 224

Irving, Kyrie, 206

Jordan, Michael, 203, 204

Joy, 105, 191, 205, 208, 211, 213, 214, 216, 217, 224–227

Kabbalah, 117

Kershaw, Clayton, 112

Kim, Chloe, 177, 203

Kinematics, 129, 131, 236

Kinesthetic, 75, 80, 233, 237, 241

Kinetic chain, 129–133, 142, 143, 176, 183, 197, 198

Kinetic chain, checkpoints, 130

Kitzman, Shawn, 114, 169

Lacrosse, 11, 199, 244

Laughing, 220

Laws of Motion, 118

Leslie, Lisa, 111

Levels of the self, 31

Lewis, Carl, 29

Life energy, 3, 37, 45, 57, 162, 243, 253

Linear motion, 118

Lloyd, Carli, 111

Lombardi, Vince, 229

Longitudinal axis, 126, 128

Love, 14, 15, 24, 26, 33, 35, 53, 54, 59, 74, 96, 105, 134, 155, 164, 181, 190, 205, 206, 209, 214, 218, 225, 231, 245, 249, 254, 261, 263

Love, Kevin, 206

Lower mind, 32, 34, 35, 37, 85

Macronutrients, 158, 160

Major league baseball, 146

Male-female healing, 139

Mandela, Nelson, 67

Martial arts, 51, 190, 199, 200

Mass, 15, 117, 123, 129, 131

Mast cells, 48, 181

McTaggart, Lynne, 117

Mechanical experts, 112

Mechanics, sports, 112, 118

Mediolateral axis, 127

Meditation, 67, 165, 218, 219, 233, 234, 259

Mental balancing, 22, 57

Mental empathy, 75

Mental health, 151, 203, 204, 206, 254

Mentors, 13, 103, 150

Meridians, 4, 18, 57, 65, 88, 89, 178, 220

Metal element, 198

Miasms, 46, 88, 178

Microbes, 19–21, 180, 181

Micronutrients, 2, 102, 157–162

Mind, 1, 4, 9, 14, 22, 31, 32, 34, 35, 37, 44, 56, 70, 71, 75, 77–79, 83, 85, 86, 88, 106, 116, 133, 134, 136, 148, 152, 155, 166, 167, 172, 174, 175, 179, 180, 182–185, 203, 204, 206–208, 211, 212, 218, 222, 224, 230, 231, 236, 242, 245, 254, 262

Minerals, 159, 162, 164, 257

Ming Men Doorway, 124, 125, 137, 138

Missing forces, 42

Molecules, 11, 97, 117, 163, 205, 216–222, 224–227, 262

Molecules of Joy, 205, 216, 224, 225, 227

Mom in the bleachers, 1, 16, 60, 68, 102, 146, 206, 229, 242

Momentum, 15, 129

Motion, 11, 15, 118, 123, 127–131, 176, 183, 199

Nadis, 18, 57, 65, 88, 128, 178, 196, 197

Nassib, Karl, 208

National Football League, 111

Natural empathy, 54, 76

Negative, 10, 21, 23, 30, 34, 36, 38, 40, 41, 43, 44, 47, 49, 57, 60, 62–64, 81, 89, 94, 95, 105, 106, 108, 117, 128, 137, 138, 148, 150–152, 161–163, 173, 174, 176, 177, 179, 181, 183, 187, 191, 194, 198, 201, 204, 207, 212, 213, 215, 220, 223, 224, 226, 232, 233, 244, 245, 247, 254

Negative charges, 57

Negative energies, 30, 41, 62, 106, 162, 163, 179, 254

Negative forces, 108, 176, 232, 233

Negative subtle charges, 40, 43, 47, 49, 57, 128

Nervous system, 38, 39, 47, 57, 158, 195–197, 221, 260

Neurochemicals, 216

Newton, Isaac, 118, 120

Nike, 203, 258

Ninth chakra, 84–86, 177, 179

Nowitzki, Dick, 111

Nutrition, 96, 147, 157–161, 163, 258, 259

Offloading, 176, 183

Oils, 95, 96, 159, 164, 186, 187, 205, 224–227

Olympics, 79, 132, 203, 204

Oneness, 117, 118, 231

Opioids, 219, 220

Osaka, Naomi, 206

Oscillations, 11

Osteocalcin, 38

Others' energies, 1, 2, 9, 11–13, 17, 23, 24, 37, 41, 45, 54, 56, 57, 60, 69, 76, 78, 88, 92, 93, 108, 129, 144, 162, 163, 172, 173, 177, 178, 182, 183, 205, 209–211, 217, 222, 223, 227, 233, 242, 261

Oxytocin, 218, 219, 226

Pain, 1, 20, 31, 45, 51, 77, 89, 92, 114, 115, 139–141, 176, 177, 180, 183, 184, 187, 204, 217, 219, 220, 226, 232

Pain-killing molecules, 219

Parallel planes, 123

Paralysis, 106, 108, 109, 112, 148, 153

Parasympathetic nervous system, 39, 197

Parents, 4, 13, 34, 40, 45, 57, 64, 103, 104, 138, 150, 246, 247, 250

Particles, 14, 73, 120

Past lives, 22, 49, 108, 125, 256

Pathways, 42, 43, 57, 128, 183, 187

Perfectionism, 4, 105, 106, 109, 112, 113, 116, 148, 153, 191, 208

Performance, 2–4, 7, 13, 15, 16, 21, 22, 25, 30, 31, 35, 36, 38, 40, 41, 52, 61, 63, 70, 75, 79, 85, 97, 99, 101, 102, 105–109, 112, 113, 116, 122, 123, 130, 131, 144, 152, 153, 162, 165, 185, 186, 189, 190, 192–194, 197, 198, 200–202, 205, 207, 209, 211, 223, 224, 233–235, 253, 260–262

Perpendicular planes, 123

Physical empathy, 54, 75, 77

Physical energy, 2, 7, 13, 23, 57, 115, 141

Physical forces, 40, 128

Pingala, 196, 197

Pitching, 1, 41, 60, 64, 112, 114, 169, 205, 207, 253, 261

Plane, 68, 122, 123, 125–128, 135, 137–140, 143, 154

Planning, 102–105, 109, 153, 189

Pleasure, 217, 218

Pleomorphism, 20

Polarity light, 72, 141, 182, 197

Polish, 102, 105, 109, 153, 192

Polyvagal nervous system, 38

Position, 15, 19, 59, 82, 114, 127, 128, 176, 209, 230

Possibilities, 56, 62, 182, 184

Post-Traumatic Stress Syndrome, 92

Post-injury, 184, 185

Power, 3, 11, 13, 16, 19, 20, 26, 29, 33, 35, 54, 56, 57, 61, 68, 71, 72, 74, 115, 118, 119, 121, 127, 129, 132, 134, 135, 148, 156, 160, 161, 174, 175, 181, 185, 191, 198, 199, 207, 231, 233, 234, 239, 245, 248, 257

Powerlessness, 107

Practice, 1, 26, 51, 67, 69–71, 74, 81, 102, 104, 105, 109, 116, 118, 119, 128, 132, 138, 152–154, 156, 160, 166, 175, 185, 192, 194, 221, 233–236, 246, 255, 257

Prayer, 3, 16, 68, 69, 92, 233, 234

Preparation, 4, 22, 23, 36, 47, 99, 113, 144, 145, 147, 148, 152, 153, 157, 167, 190, 201

Presence element, 134

Probabilities, 182

Procrastination, 106–109, 112, 148, 153

Programming, 9, 95, 97, 156, 160, 166, 185, 263

Programs, 16, 46, 53, 59, 61, 85, 138, 147, 149, 150, 154, 155, 173, 225, 262

Prophecy, 54, 76

Protection, 176, 183, 202

Proteins, 158, 161, 163, 164

Psychic, 13, 75–78, 176, 177, 179, 180, 207, 235, 236, 245

Psychic surgery, 176, 177, 179, 180

Psychological issues, 165, 208

Quanta/quantum, 11, 13–16, 27, 73, 113–116, 117–121, 129, 144, 172, 182

Quantum fields, 172

Quantum fluctuations, 73, 182

Quantum laws, 118

Quantum physics, 13, 114, 116, 144

Quick Absentee Healing, 94

Racquetball, 199

Random Event Generators, 117

Reconditioning, 176, 184

Regression, 22, 35, 69, 86

Reiki, 3, 92, 93, 258

Reincarnation, 33

Relational empathy, 54, 75, 76

Religion, 68, 70, 234, 248

Resonance, 19, 21

Reward molecules, 217

Rife Universal Microscope, 19

Rife, Royal Raymond, 19

Rotation, 127, 154, 266

Rugby, 199

Running, 26, 59, 119, 120, 131, 134, 146, 154, 161, 200, 218, 219, 246

Sabotage, 85, 108

Sadness, 213, 214, 225

Sagittal axis, 126, 127

Sagittal plane, physical, 122, 125, 138

Sagittal plane, subtle, 122, 127, 138

Sale, Chris, 112

Samadhi, 175, 199, 231, 234

Sanborn, Kate, 145, 146

Scalar waves, 15, 72–74, 84

Schizophrenia, 217

Second chakra, 75, 137, 163, 222, 249

Second Law of Acceleration, 120

Sequencing, 22, 91, 119–121, 129, 135, 142, 154

Serotonin, 221, 222, 226

Serotonin Syndrome, 222

Seventh chakra, 76, 222, 248, 249

Shamanism, 76

Shame, 44, 64, 161, 177, 225

Shinrin-yoku, *see* forest bathing

Shock, 39, 40, 46, 51, 63, 108, 176, 179, 183, 187, 202, 250

Shock bubble, 40, 46, 51, 108, 176, 179, 183, 187, 250

Sixth chakra, 80, 219, 247, 249

Skating, 22, 125, 128, 199

Skiing, 75, 199, 200, 207, 218

Sleep, 12, 147, 159, 165–167, 189, 190, 192, 208, 218, 221, 233, 243, 258, 259

Sleep exercises, 165–167

Snowboarding, 199, 203

Soccer, 104, 111, 176, 190, 198, 200, 229, 245

Softball, 3, 12, 26, 199

Soul, 22, 31–35, 37, 40, 44, 46, 53, 56, 60, 77, 78, 83, 86, 88, 105, 106, 121, 125, 135, 136, 139, 140, 148, 155, 164, 171, 172, 174, 175, 177, 179, 182, 204, 205, 215, 221, 222, 254, 256

Soul issues, 40, 46

Sound, 11, 18, 20, 57, 59, 86, 118, 121, 134, 157, 162, 172, 174, 181, 195, 198, 200, 234, 235, 256

Sound element, 134

Sound, and chakras, 18, 59, 86

Source, 10, 33, 53, 64, 108, 133, 182, 211, 214, 220, 233

Speed, 15, 19, 72, 85, 114, 119, 131, 142, 156, 165, 199, 253

Speed of light, 15, 72, 85, 119

Spin, 11, 15, 19, 125, 128

Spine, 15, 22, 37, 56, 80, 115, 128, 130, 139–142, 154, 197, 215, 216, 221

Spirals, 56, 60, 106, 144

Spirit-mundane healing, 140

Spiritual forces, 41

Spiritual guides, 24, 70, 149, 152, 243, 256

Spiritual qualities, 73, 125

Spiritual teams, 155

Spirituality, 54, 68, 70, 248

Sports, psychologists, 105, 155, 204, 254

Sports, trainers, 1, 2, 4, 13, 243

Squares, 144

Squash, 199

Stability, 4, 129, 162

Star element, 134

Stokjko, Elvis, 51

Stone element, 134

Stones, 96, 181, 186, 187, 257

Strength building, 22

Stress, 9, 22, 36, 38–40, 43, 44, 46, 47, 49, 89, 92, 149, 159, 180, 187, 189, 194–196, 206, 208, 218–220, 222, 255, 259

Stress hormones, 38

Stressor, 36, 38, 40, 46, 47

Stretching, 22

Stuck points, 42, 43

Subatomic quanta/particles, 11

Subconscious self, 85

Subluminal level, 85, 132

Subtle elements, 132, 134, 180, 182, 183, 190, 193, 198–200, 202, 232, 233

Subtle energy, 2, 3, 7, 10, 17–19, 43, 44, 52, 57, 68, 69, 76, 112, 129, 136, 141, 144, 153, 157, 172, 173, 175–177, 187, 197, 209, 218, 222, 227, 257

Subtle energy anatomy, 7, 17, 44, 52

Subtle energy tools, 10, 52, 69

Subtle fields, 92

Subtle organs, 17

Success, 4, 17, 20, 24, 44, 57, 59, 61–63, 65, 78, 79, 101, 102, 104–107, 109, 121, 135, 139, 144–149, 151, 155, 162, 164, 165, 191, 192, 194, 203, 204, 244, 249, 261

Superstring theory, 117

Supraluminal level, 85

Surfing, 199

Sushumna, 128, 196, 197

Swimming, 64, 76, 199, 200

Sympathetic nervous system, 39, 47, 197

Team members, 149–151, 218

Template, 177, 179

Tennis, 12, 16, 17, 67, 74, 120, 154, 170, 171, 173, 189, 199, 200, 206, 257

Tenth chakra, 76, 80, 84–86, 130, 137, 142, 156, 193

Thalamus, 39

Theory of resonance, 21

Theory of transformation, 21

Third chakra, 35, 75, 104, 137, 245, 249

Third Law of Counterforce, 120

Thoughts, 34, 60, 63, 65, 75, 76, 96, 115, 117, 135, 157, 161–163, 167, 177, 198, 202, 204, 205, 212, 233, 235, 245

Three Axes of Movement, 126

Three Cardinal Planes, 122, 123, 125, 127, 135, 138

Tommy John surgery, 101, 170, 219

Track, 15, 25, 29, 52, 119, 142, 161, 177, 207, 223

Traditional Chinese medicine, 57, 124, 137

Transverse plane, physical, 125

Transverse plane, subtle, 125

Trauma, 4, 22, 33, 35–39, 46, 48, 49, 56, 108, 187, 194, 255, 260, 263

Trauma model, 46

Triangles, 144

Trivedi, Mahendra Kumar (Guruji), 16

Tummo, 116

Twelfth chakra, 54

Uncertainty Principle, 14

Unconscious Self, 85

Ups and downs, 4, 25, 77, 99, 104, 203, 209, 219, 230, 251

Vagus nerve, 38, 39, 57, 194, 195, 197

Velocity, 29, 120, 129, 131, 142, 144, 169, 207

Verbal force, 41

Vibration, 11, 12, 19, 20, 31

Vibrational remedies, 3, 7, 22, 69, 89, 147, 153, 171, 190, 201, 202, 224, 257

Virtual light, 73, 85, 141, 182, 197

Virtual light, for healing, 73, 182

Visualization, 69, 79, 147, 150, 151, 184, 192, 260

Vitamins, 158, 159, 162, 224

Vivaxis, 119, 132–134, 233

Void, 26, 73, 198, 199

Volleyball, 3, 25, 42, 200

Walking, 24, 104, 125, 136, 154, 170, 182, 183, 192, 200, 211, 222, 224, 239

Water element, 134

Water, importance, 95

Water, programming, 95–97, 156, 160, 164, 180

Waves, 14, 15, 59, 72–74, 83, 84, 116, 120, 165, 166

Weight, 15, 37, 119, 129, 144, 158, 160

Weightlifting, 44

Wilson, Russell, 145

Wolfskins, 115, 116

Wooden, John, vii

Woods, Tiger, 64

Workout programs, 154

Workouts, 10, 37, 113, 129, 147, 153–155, 158, 220, 232, 236, 238, 254, 258

Worthiness molecules, 221

Wounding, 179

Yoga, 51, 194, 218, 220, 221, 257, 260

To Write to the Author

If you wish to contact the author or would like more information about this book, please write to the author in care of Llewellyn Worldwide and we will forward your request. Both the author and the publisher appreciate hearing from you and learning of your enjoyment of this book and how it has helped you. Llewellyn Worldwide cannot guarantee that every letter written to the author can be answered, but all will be forwarded. Please write to:

Cyndi Dale
℅ Llewellyn Worldwide
2143 Wooddale Drive
Woodbury, MN 55125-2989

Please enclose a self-addressed stamped envelope for reply or $1.00 to cover costs. If outside the USA, enclose an international postal reply coupon.

Many of Llewellyn's authors have websites with additional information and resources. For more information, please visit our website:

WWW.LLEWELLYN.COM